EXERCISING VALUES
PAMELA DAVENPORT

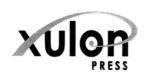

Copyright © 2011 by Pamela Davenport

EXERCISING VALUES
by Pamela Davenport

Printed in the United States of America

ISBN 9781613791226

All rights reserved solely by the author. The author guarantees all contents are original and do not infringe upon the legal rights of any other person or work. No part of this book may be reproduced in any form without the permission of the author. The views expressed in this book are not necessarily those of the publisher.

Unless otherwise indicated, Bible quotations are taken from THE HOLY BIBLE, NEW INTERNATIONAL VERSION®, NIV®. Copyright © 1973, 1978, 1984, 2011 by Biblica, Inc.™ Used by permission. All rights reserved worldwide.

www.xulonpress.com

FORWARD

No one goes to tea parties anymore. At age four, my mom took me to a swimming pool and tried to coax me into putting my head under the water. She suggested we have a tea party on the bottom of the pool. So I took a deep breath and sank down so I could pretend to eat cookies and pass tea cups. Years later, I competed on my high school and college swim teams; so I guess it must have worked. More amazing to me is that I still remember that summer tea party. Frankly, I recall thinking it was pretty silly, even at the time.

Maybe you remember another tea party. Do you recall watching the children in Mary Poppins enjoying a tea party on the ceiling? Laughing made them levitate into the air. When our children reminisce about their time with us, we want them to remember at least one episode of good-natured, uncontrollable laughter. We're going to aim high in this program: endeavoring to teach good character and instill a love of movement that will lead to a lifetime of physical fitness. While on this important and noble quest, it's okay to have a lot of fun. Exercising Values isn't a to do list meant to be checked off. It's a party. It's running, jumping, laughing fun. Enjoy!

ACKNOWLEDGMENTS

Exercising Values has been a family affair with my husband, Doug, reading the stories from great literature, my daughter Jennifer suggesting stories to include; Tiffany, Skyler, Hilary, and Kian helping to promote the book and most of all, my oldest son, Dane, doing all the web design and set up, illustrating the workouts, and joining me in the mastermind group Ryan Lee provided. I love you all and appreciate your support and hard work.

I home educated my children using the educational program of the Advanced Training Institute. I learned the value of a systematic character training program from them. They are a great resource for additional character curriculum. If you are considering home education, I highly recommend that you look into their program. I am very grateful to Bill Gothard and everyone connected to ATI for all the training and support they provided our family.

I owe a debt of gratitude to Vince DelMonte who suggested I attend one of Ryan Lee's events where Ryan encouraged me to write what was close to my heart. Ryan and his sidekick Geo Diovanni as well as the mastermind group members provided a lot of advice and direction. So I thank each of you for helping me get started. I also want to thank Christopher Guerriero who also counseled me early on and was in fact one of the first people to express a lot of enthusiasm for the work before it was even written. Tom Bird and his authors group in Sedona gave me encouragement and a great place to push through to finish the book.

Many friends and family members also gave me words of encouragement and I'm grateful for each one of you. Many friends also lent me their children to test the exercises and I want to thank them and their children for their enthusiastic support and helpful feedback.

One special friend that stands out is Angie Dasbauch. Her interest and enthusiasm for the work was a source of encouragement and much needed practical help as she advised me on the editing process.

Finally, and most importantly I am grateful to you, the reader who has invested in this book as a way of investing in your children and their future. I am excited to have you experience greater health, a happier family, and children who will exhibit wisdom and depth of character in the days to come. Thank you for your trust and commitment.

CHAPTER ONE
RAISING CHILDREN IS SERIOUS BUSINESS

It's not really a conspiracy but it might as well be. There are so many forces in today's world, each with their own agenda, vying for the allegiance of our children. We have to be proactive to keep the influence that used to be the birthright of every parent. The problem for busy parents has never been a lack of concern or caring, but rather a lack of a blueprint or even a place to start.

Exercising Values provides that place to start. I want to help insure that your voice will at least be among the voices that your child will hear and remember today. The voice that only has their best interests at heart is yours and you need to make it understood.

Anything can be lost in just one generation if parents fail to pass it on. Sadly, at times our lives can get so hectic that we might find ourselves giving more thought to what we will have for lunch today than how we plan to invest in our children's future. It's not your fault. Providing just for their physical needs via a paycheck can be so exhausting that little energy is left to think about the rest. It's easy to feel overwhelmed. Because I know you want to do more for your children, I want to give you the tools you'll need.

The Timeless Values of Health, Character and Family Togetherness

We all know that the world our children will raise their own children in will be vastly different than the one we live in today. With the inevitable change driven by technology and other forces, we need to identify what core values and habits we insist on passing on. We are in effect drawing a line in the sand and saying these truths have timeless value and we will make them a part of the fabric of our children's early years. Building health, character, and family togetherness is the place to start and increases your chances of achieving any additional goals you set.

I recently watched an engaging talk by JJ Abrams on Ted.com. He showed a clip from Jaws where Roy Scheider is sitting at the dinner table with his young son of three or four. Roy's character is obviously stressed and deep in thought as he contemplates his shark problem.

As he wrings his hands and covers his face, his young son copies every nuance of his father's body language. Perhaps not as shocking as the scene where the shark explodes out of the water, it is every bit as gripping. It should be equally terrifying if we are not confident of the example we are setting for our observant children. But we are not the only ones that they are watching and emulating.

Identifying the "Sharks" in our Midst

Advancing technologies have made it possible for us to surround ourselves with whatever information we wish. We have more choices than ever before and the quality of our character will drive those choices. Great teachers and interesting lecturers are now within reach via the internet. But we've had the technology to surround ourselves with quality information for years. Its called television and we all know how that has turned out.

Years ago one MTV executive was quoted as saying "At MTV we don't shoot for the fourteen year olds, we own them." Does that presumption enrage you as it does me? Likewise we are doubly enraged by the exploitation of children on pornographic sites. Most technology can be used for good or evil.

As they grow up, our children will need to discern not just between good and evil but between mediocrity and the truly valuable. Of all the resources available to children the one we really don't want to waste is our own ability to influence them for good. We can't protect them simply by limiting access to bad content. They must be taught principles so they can evaluate whether or not they are "setting evil in front of their eyes"; something the Bible urged us not to do long before a television set or computer screen was an option.

In Jaws, the father paused when he realized that his son was copying him and he asked him for a hug. The son asked why and he replied, "because I need one." We have our own daily sharks that distract us and make us unavailable to our children. This makes our children unable to give us that needed hug. But they are still observing us. Maybe it inspires them to try to be like us and maybe it drives them to be anything but like us. Either way, our actions and attitudes impact theirs.

Exercising Values will help you be intentional about the example you set for your children. It requires fifteen minutes a day to specifically model and teach health and good character. You will forge a bond with your children by consistently giving them this time and attention.

With all the forces trying to lure your child, purposely exerting your own influence may seem like a futile effort. Maybe even like a drop in the ocean. The impact of small but consistent actions are more like drops of water striking the same spot on a rock. They will eventually split that rock apart. Exercising Values is focused on excellent character development and excellent physical fitness. That's our rock. If we repeat our influence on these two areas on a daily basis then change will occur.

Setting the Bar High for our Children

That "A" you hope to see on a report card stands for excellence. We want our children to be excellent. More than that, we want it to be in ways that matter for their well-being and influence on the world. I don't pretend to have all the answers when it comes to parenting but I am very confident that this program will aid it's users in reaching their goals for their children.

Exercising Values is modeled on the Biblical injunction to give you and your children a hope and a future. I invite you to read this book and try the program for a month. See if it's a good fit for your family. If you join the battle for your child's direction in life, I believe you will win. The MTV executive was wrong, they don't own anyone, least of all your child.

The play on words of Exercising Values should have given you some idea that physical fitness is one of the three legs holding up our stool. The second is character or being able to discern and do what's right, even when it is costly to do so. While you are doing your workouts together, you will also be introducing various character qualities and talking about their value. The final leg is strong family bonds that come from regularly doing something worthwhile together as a family.

Amazingly, through the power of consistent action, we are going to accomplish all this in as little as fifteen minutes a day. With the foundation of this minimum daily requirement, you can build from there; exposing your children to all the experiences you think are important for them.

Family Routines Ensure What's Most Important Gets Done

The Journal of Family Psychology reviewed fifty years of research on family routines. The overwhelming consensus was that routines help children feel secure, strengthen family bonds, improve health, and lead to greater productivity. It even enhances intellect by stimulating both right and left brain activity.

What you will readily observe will confirm these benefits. It is not something you will need to force on your children. Instead, your children will remind you it's time for Exercising Values because they look forward to it each day.

Do you remember reading the story about the world-renowned violinist Joshua Bell, who stood alone and played in a crowded train station in Washington D.C.? His beautiful music flowed to all around him but very few seemed to even notice this remarkable event. In a different venue, these same people might have paid thousands of dollars to hear this same music played by this same genius. On this day, it went largely unnoticed. The few who dropped a bit of money for the performer collectively didn't even leave him enough for a simple meal.

The crowd in the train station missed the chance of a lifetime. It was a free concert just for them hosted by a virtuoso. Consumed by their own errands and distracting thoughts they never stopped to appreciate the gift he gave them that day. Some opportunities truly are once in a lifetime. Time with our children is also a once in a lifetime opportunity but it too, is easy to take for granted.

The urgency of our schedules and to-do lists can blind us to special, fleeting moments. That laughing baby that was so popular on YouTube for a while became popular because of his innocent, enthusiastic entrancement with the present moment; a lost art for most grown-ups. We like to be reminded of what it feels like to be delighted; to simply throw back our heads and laugh uncontrollably. Explore your daily life for these untapped and unnoticed resources, potential, and gifts.

As an experienced family counselor and the mother of six children, I would hate to see you miss any opportunities to put a solid foundation under your children. I want you to pass on to them what you value most. The truth is, it is easy to be distracted, tired and busy and not realize what we are missing or how quickly time is passing.

There is a scene in the movie Steel Magnolias where the diabetic daughter is talking to her mother about her decision to conceive a child at the risk of her own life. She says that she "would rather have thirty minutes of wonderful than a lifetime of nothing special." Fail to plan how you will weave what is most important in life into your daily schedule and soon enough you'll have lived "a lifetime of nothing special".

I believe Exercising Values can help you implement your good intentions. It only asks for fifteen minutes of your busy day; just long enough to stop to listen to a virtuoso or to laugh with all your might. During this brief time, on the physical side, you will invest in your own health and fitness. You will burn fat and encourage your children to be lean, strong and healthy. You will teach character qualities such as diligence, enthusiasm, hospitality, and loyalty in a way that your children will enjoy and remember.

Just the simple act of scheduling daily time with your children to do Exercising Values will send them the strong message that they are important to you. They will have attention from you that they can count on. No one has to sit still. You are getting a workout and your kids are getting to play with you, learn from you, and receive lots of love and affirmation. As you work and play together, you will share many memories and grow closer. The quality of your influence on them will grow.

The Amazing Synergy of Teaching Fitness and Character Together

Much of the power and effectiveness of this system comes from teaching character and physical fitness together. Children are naturally going to be more receptive to what you are saying when they are moving and playing with you rather than being forced to sit still. Would you want to only hear about character when you are in trouble; like having your boss ask you why you are lazy or hard to get along with? Of course not. Children are the same way. Being positive is important and timing is everything.

Children are not the only ones who benefit from focused attention on character. You, too, will develop as a person. Then, by improving your own character, you will be a more effective role-model for your children. Character and fitness reinforce each other causing everyone to improve. You may even lose weight or get in better shape because of your own reflections about diligence or enthusiasm.

In quieter moments, one of the best ways to reinforce the character lesson is through classic children's literature. Great literature is great mostly because it wrestles in some way with choices involving character. I have chosen each story because it illuminates the character quality of the week.

Share these specially selected stories at bedtime, while you rest after the workout or whenever you have some leisure time. Wonderful memories and strong family bonds will be created. You will have carved out some pleasant, stress-free moments in your day.

As a convenience, a recorded version of the story is available through my website: www.exercisingvalues.com. It can be played over and over to reinforce the character quality they have just learned. It's wonderful to listen together but by having them recorded your children can have access to them even when you are unavailable. Alternatively, you can find and read these recommended stories aloud to your children.

These stories are the perfect adjunct to the daily exercise and character program. They will ensure that your children will later reflect deeply upon these new concepts which were brought to their attention briefly but repeatedly while you exercised together.

In the next few chapters we will look more closely at the three main areas that Exercising Values is designed to improve. They are:

1. Family Physical Fitness

2. Behavior through Character Education and Development

3. Family Bonding and Togetherness

The power of working on all three of these goals at the same time is tremendous. The sum is indeed greater than the parts. This is due to the power of association. You will be connecting good health habits and sound character to warm and fun family times.

How many people learned to hate sports because of the memory of being picked last in gym class or otherwise feeling awkward in front of their peers? Don't leave it to chance that your children will think exercise is pleasant and something they want to do. Create the best environment possible to learn the values and the habits you believe are in their best interest.

You will be helping your children to see that you value physical fitness and want them to take care of their bodies. Your encouragement will help them see themselves as physically capable. Their happy memories with you will set them up for a lifetime of healthy choices. This active, fun context will open your children's hearts to what you want to teach them.

The Power of Scheduling Time to Spend with your Family

Regularly scheduled time together is beneficial in and of itself. A study conducted at BYU and published in July, 2010 analyzed 148 published longitudinal studies to access the factors that contribute to longevity. They found that social interaction is more important to longevity than exercise and twice as important as avoiding obesity. They even found that low social interaction had a similar impact on lifespan as being an alcoholic or smoking 15 cigarettes a day. They determined that having social ties with friends, family, and others can improve our odds of survival by fifty percent.

We live in an age when children are often connecting to others through machines rather than through face to face interactions. We don't yet know the impact of that on their health and well-being. Until we know more on that subject, we can know that a lack of social relationships is a health risk and that strong family ties help prevent it.

CHAPTER TWO
A ROADMAP FOR ENHANCING THE PHYSICAL FITNESS OF YOUR FAMILY

You've probably heard the saying popularized by Stephan Covey that when you are climbing a ladder it's important to know that it is leaning against the right wall. The "right wall" for our children includes physical health and well-being and values that will guide them to make good choices and decisions. Athletics has long been looked up to as a character-building experience. Many people will sacrifice time and money to give their children the advantages of being involved in sports.

Exercise promotes health, prevents obesity, relieves stress, and is a vehicle for fun. It has a place in every child's life and their first and favorite coach should be you. This should ring true whether or not you think you are raising a potential superstar.

The Pros and Cons to Organized Athletics and Team Sports for Children

Organized athletics are great but not the only way to get your children to be active. Being pulled in many directions, families that love sports and athletics want to find more ways to enjoy being active together. Sometimes it feels like something is missing.

I've seen harried parents plop down at a soccer game after managing the quick pre-game snack and car pool. While their children dash back and forth across the field, they sit and sit some more. That's fine. They are there to cheer and show support. But I believe that if earlier that day they too had engaged in some vigorous physical activity that they would have arrived at the game with more energy. Then they could relax and enjoy themselves more. They could also share in their child's enthusiasm for sport on a different level.

In addition, their child would take the memory of that family time with them onto the field, including the associated character lesson. Think of the attitude problems coaches sometimes have to deal with suddenly disappearing, as the young athletes strive to exhibit traits like diligence, kindness, and perseverance. Parents are in the unique position of being able to link physical fitness and the sense of being loved and noticed with good character in their children's minds. It is quite likely that their children will continue throughout life to enjoy sports and to feel like an important part of the family.

My own six children have been intensely involved in gymnastics and basketball as well as having some exposure to swim teams, soccer, golf, triathlon, baseball, and track. I know all too well the pressure these sports can put on families as they build their schedules, free time, and even meal times and vacations around them. I also know the joy of seeing children find a sport they love, reach goals and feel successful. Exercising with the family at a young age can plant the seeds to more serious athletic pursuits or just lay the foundation for less structured life time fitness.

As your children grow they will develop their own interests and special abilities so much so that you might not be able to keep up with them. Although I may love running, you are never going to see me running full speed at a vault as all of my children have done. Twirl around a high bar like my son, Kian, does? Of course not. It'll never be anything but a spectator sport for me; a chance for me to see my son excel at gymnastics and to be amazed by what he can do. He puts in many hours of practice now but the foundation was laid when he learned to love movement as a young child.

Knowing that you had even a small role in fostering your child's achievements will be deeply satisfying. Simple athletic training will open many options for them in the future. In this book, I will teach you how to teach your children these basic athletic skills. They will bring you joy both now and in the future.

Finding Time to Keep Fit as a Busy Parent

You may also have your own hobbies that you want to pursue. Maybe you love golf, tennis, or participating in races. I'm a triathlete and have been able to travel and compete as part of Team USA. I'm grateful for the chance to represent my country and meet people from all over the world. In this season of life, I am able to take advantage of these opportunities.

When I had six children twelve and younger, it was a different story. My workouts almost always included the children and were usually done at home. As they have grown, we continue to enjoy the occasional run or game of tennis together. We have happy memories of the physical activities we did when they were young which transitioned into the sports they enjoy today. By staying active with your children you can "hold your place in line" until you come into a season of life that allows you more time for your own athletic pursuits.

I realize that the lifestyles of the parents who use Exercising Values will vary greatly. Some of you are home educating families who are incorporating Exercising Values into your physical education and literature curriculum. Others are single parents juggling family and at least one job, sometimes two or more. Still others are two career families that sometimes only see each other coming and going.

Whatever your circumstances, Exercising Values will help you protect your own health through enhanced fitness. In addition, you can dramatically improve your communication with your children, earn their respect, and guide their lives toward healthy attitudes and behaviors. By participating with your children in Exercising Values on a regular basis, you become their role model and their guide.

Let's face it; to truly influence our children toward health and well-being they need to see us practicing solid health habits like exercise ourselves. And if in the process, we shed a few pounds, look and feel better, and have an abundance of energy; then we'll just have to live with these side effects of loving our kids so much. Motivated to help them, we finally take action on our own health goals and everyone is better off.

Stemming the Tide of Childhood Obesity

Not every family aspires to have their children active in sports, however, we all know that exercise has many health promoting benefits. If this describes your family, you may be looking for guidance on how to be active together in order to stay healthy. I understand that you lead full lives so I've kept the time commitment to a minimum without sacrificing results.

The staggering rise in childhood obesity alerts all of us to get involved where young children's health is concerned. Anyone would shudder to learn that the Center for Disease Control estimates that half of all children and adolescents in the United States are now clinically obese. As a certified personal trainer, I've worked with countless families to avoid this tragedy in their family and I'd like to share my expertise with your family as well.

The short effective workouts in Exercising Values can be done together as a family and because they rely on bodyweight are suitable for children as well as adults. They will help both parents and children control their weight and build the strength and coordination that is useful in everyday activities. Designed to be fun and educational they can be the foundation for many happy childhood memories as well as a solid foundation for a lifetime of fitness.

The Importance of Getting Started Right Away

Confession time. Over the years, I have bought programs and books that I thought would benefit my children and then I never actually got around to using them. I imagine that this is pretty common in today's busy world. So before we get started, let's take a minute to commit to beginning and finishing the first month's program.

Teaching character while promoting physical fitness leads to the long held ideal of the sound mind in a sound body. We don't want to neglect either one in our quest to raise extraordinary children. So just commit to trying this formula for at least a month and see the difference it makes in your children's behavior and happiness.

Don't worry about mastering every detail or being perfect. Don't procrastinate; instead choose a start date and then stick to it. Announce it to your kids and they'll help you get started. Getting started can be the hardest part so ignore distractions and begin.

That may mean turning off the television, phone, email, etc. Fifteen minutes is all you need. These short bursts will create momentum and soon a new habit will be formed. Performing the workout and reinforcing the character quality is the task you want to complete each day.

When you do get it done, feel great. When you don't, don't criticize yourself or worse, blame each other. Just restart the next day and realize change is a process that may have a lot of ups and downs. Don't be discouraged. You are moving in the right direction.

You are in the process of taking control of an important aspect of your life. You will be improving your own fitness and that of your children while teaching an important aspect of character. Each day, you have time set aside to enjoy each other's company. Better food choices will naturally follow to support your new activity level. Your children will thrive because they are receiving the gift of your attention and time.

If you are passionate and excited about growing closer as a family while pursuing health and character, then you absolutely will be successful. Give it the priority in your schedule that it deserves. This program is all about small steps taken consistently to build big results over time. Be enthusiastic and create some fun and your children won't be able to wait to get started each day.

When the inevitable interruptions, both great and small, come; just remember that they are a normal part of life. They do not necessarily mean you can't persist with the program to which you've committed. As beloved basketball coach, John Wooden, once said, "Don't let what you cannot do interfere with what you can do." Keeping to this simple routine may actually make it easier to get through the disruptive event. But when you must set your routine aside for a short time, also decide on the time you will begin again. Perfection is never necessary with this program. Commitment is.

Planning Extraordinary Weekends

Weekend fun is part of the Exercising Values plan. On the weekend, we have more time to spend together. We have been presenting our short character lessons during the fifteen minute workouts that take place on week days. During this time we also need to build excitement for Game Day which is on Saturday or whatever day parents are off work. Game Day provides a built in reminder to make each weekend special.

Many people gain weight on the weekends. Focus on the fun and not the food and this won't happen to you. Avoid stuffing negative feelings down with food or treating food as a reward for your week of work. Instead create positive feelings by spending time with your loved ones and let those good times be your reward.

The seeds of emotional eating in adulthood are sown in childhood. Rescue yourself from this negative learned behavior while preventing its future practice in your children. Whereas others may always include junk foods with leisure times, you can choose equally enjoyable but healthy foods.

Game day gives you a chance to spend extended time with your children and they will look forward to it whether you can spare an hour or the whole day. Besides the routine fitness activities, you may also want to come up with some special events to add some variety. When my oldest children were still very small, we started a tradition that we still do today. This is despite the fact that five of my six children are now old enough to vote.

Our family loves to follow the Olympics and I knew that that would involve a lot of sitting around watching television. I wanted a way to balance that with activity so we instituted the Olympic Challenge.

Every Olympics, from the time the torch is lit at the opening ceremony until it is extinguished at the closing ceremony, our family competes to see who can do the most push-ups, jumps with a jump rope, and some agreed upon abdominal exercise. Some years, as they have grown older, we have also added miles ran. We award gold, silver, and bronze in these individual events as well as an all-around award.

We post our daily progress on the refrigerator so we always know where we stand. Those standings have motivated many a late night push-up that otherwise would never have occurred. Often I was the one doing them, trying to keep up with a seven year old or a teenager.

So the take home message is: fitness with your family is fun. A little friendly competition can be motivating from time to time especially when your children have a chance to win. Copy this idea or find your own excuse for a fitness celebration. Occasionally, no matter how great the program, doing things a bit differently for a time will give you a break. The coverage of the Olympics usually features stories about how various athletes overcame obstacles. Incorporate these into your character lessons.

When she was about ten years old my daughter, Tiffany's favorite story was about renowned Olympic track star, Wilma Rudolph. Wilma braved poverty, illness and discrimination to become a national phenomena. She overcame the adversity of being born prematurely, of having a long string of childhood illnesses including measles, mumps, double pneumonia, scarlet fever, and chicken pox. Then she contracted polio and the doctor said that she would never walk again.

She was the twentieth of twenty-two children but her hard-working mother refused to accept this diagnosis and found time to go to great lengths to get her the medical attention she needed. Wilma Rudolph not only walked; eventually she became one of the most celebrated athletes of all time. She won four Olympic medals for track. Among her many honors, she was inducted into the Olympic Hall of Fame in 1983.

Tiffany admired Wilma's determination and loved the fact that her many brothers and sisters were such an encouragement to her. She read the biography about her over and over again. Look beyond your own family for character role models and you will find them.

My two oldest sons had Michael Jordan all over their room as young boys. The story goes that he was passed over early in his high school basketball career only to later become a sports legend. Children are bolstered by examples of people who don't give up . They will notice if you faithfully continue this program. Think about Wilma's mother when you are tempted to give up. Can you even imagine meeting the needs of twenty-two children? I can't.

Ten Suggestions for Building a Memorable Weekend

1. Look at a photo album together and try to do the first active thing you see. So, if a photo of someone in a baseball cap shows up, you head out the door to play ball. If you see a picture at the beach, you at least try to go swimming. If it happens to be a picture with a pile of leaves; time to rake some up and jump in the middle. No photo album? Use a magazine.

2. Have a picnic. Don't let bad weather stop you. It can be just as much fun to have a picnic indoors. Associate this fun activity with healthy food choices. A lot of lifelong damaging emotional eating can be prevented now by establishing healthy foods as your children's comfort foods.

3. Go for a walk. There is something about walking together that makes people also talk and share things they might not otherwise have shared. It gives them your uninterrupted attention. It doesn't have to all be serious talk. While you are walking you could create a story together. Each family member gets to add one sentence at a time. These stories can obviously be quite funny. At times, they can also be insightful as to your children's interests and concerns.

4. Jump rope. It helps prevent osteoporosis and it is lots of fun. Just fifty small jumps a day can help keep the minerals in your bones as you age.

5. Go skating, bowling, or miniature golfing.

6. Camp in the backyard. Look at the stars. Drink hot chocolate, hot lemonade, or maybe it's time for that tea party we talked about. Meteor showers in the middle of the night aren't convenient but they are memorable.

7. Listen to the story from Exercising Values together. You may want to get one of the additional complete books and listen to the whole thing together over several days.

8. All traditional sports fit in well on the weekend. Play golf, tennis, basketball, baseball, or go skiing or fishing. Expose your children to lots of sports and spend some time teaching them your favorite one.

9. Dance around or otherwise act silly, take some pictures and send them to grandma. I'm a grandmother now so I can say on good authority these photos will be cherished.

10. Play tag. You'll be surprised by how much exercise you'll get.

This is just a list to get you started. I'm sure you'll have lots to add. As your children get older, they will enjoy coming up with suggestions for family activities. Listen to them and help them to own this family time.

Spending quality time with your family is a great stress reliever which in turn leads to better weight control. Some of the above activities will only take fifteen minutes and others might take all day. Let your choices reflect what else you have going on that weekend. Don't skip it altogether when you have a particularly full weekend. Game day should be fun for you too, so keep it simple.

I know you want to pass on the best of what you have to offer to your children and enrich their life with your own. You want to inspire your children to greatness or at least impress upon them that they have gifts to give. Health and good character will help these gifts grow and help your child reach their potential.

Exercising Values is designed to help you equip them to excel. Set the bar high by exposing them to physical fitness and great literature and then let them know that you believe in them. Your investment in them will pay off. Your child is your magnum opus, the best work of your life.

CHAPTER THREE
INSTILLING GOOD CHARACTER LEADS TO WELL-BEHAVED CHILDREN

Our children's physical well-being is only part of our deep concern for them. We also want to see them prepared to make good choices in life and to exhibit great character. It also warms our hearts when others comment on how well-behaved our children are. When behavior stems from the child actually understanding the desirability of various aspects of good character, then good behavior becomes second nature. Parents can relax when they see their children adopting appropriate behavior as their own.

Parents striving for these ideals are swimming up stream in our culture. The statistics on youth moral decay are unfortunately every bit as alarming as those on their physical decline. A recent British report issued by their Department of Children found from their survey of 11,000 fifteen and sixteen year old students an increase in the acceptability of lying, speeding and underage drinking. According to several United States studies lying, stealing and cheating are on the rise both in schools and in the work place. It's gravely concerning that these behaviors aren't just occurring but they are increasingly seen as acceptable.

News stories abound of children being victimized by bullies. Some of this is occurring online and some in person. One expert calls it "the vulture culture". Parents are being forced to teach their children how to protect themselves. All parents are responsible to teach their children not to behave in a threatening or disparaging way to others. The time to teach these things is long before a problem arises.

Before you let all this discourage you, take heart in knowing that studies have also shown that today's youth also have an amazingly strong altruistic bent. They want to make the world a better place for others. When you take the time to define good character and encourage its practice, you give your children something to which to aspire. You inspire them to be people who will make a difference in this world. You give them something they are looking for: guidance.

There are resources available to help you expand on what Exercising Values introduces. Over the past decade hundreds of cities across the United States and around the world have designated themselves to be character cities. Leaders in these cities work to encourage citizens to focus on the forty-nine character qualities listed below. They even post them on billboards and include them in city newsletters.

What you begin in your home with your own children is part of a larger effort to build a community of character. There are resources available to help you expand on what Exercising Values introduces. But no one is in a better position to teach these timeless truths to your children than you are.

Identifying Timeless Character Qualities Worth Passing On

Though it is true that character is caught as well as taught; a well thought out plan to teach values goes a long way to ensuring that we are teaching the things we aspire to model for our children. Our ladder will be leaning against the right wall. So each week, a character quality is presented that we can explore and practice each day.

Here is a list to get you started:

Alertness, Attentiveness, Availability, Boldness, Cautiousness, Compassion, Contentment, Creativity, Decisiveness, Deference, Dependability, Determination, Diligence, Discernment, Discretion, Endurance, Enthusiasm, Faith, Flexibility, Forgiveness, Generosity, Gentleness, Gratefulness, Honor, Hospitality, Humility, Initiative, Joyfulness, Justice, Kindness, Love, Loyalty, Meekness, Obedience, Orderliness, Patience, Persuasiveness, Punctuality, Resourcefulness, Respectfulness, Responsibility, Security, Self-control, Sensitivity, Sincerity, Thoughtfulness, Thoroughness, Thriftiness, Tolerance, Truthfulness, Virtue, and Wisdom.

You may think of others that you'd like to add but this list is a good place to start. Having a list will help you to take action and will ensure that you are introducing the concept of each character quality to your children. Most people naturally value one aspect of good character over another so without a comprehensive list they might overlook teaching an essential concept. While some people are more naturally orderly, punctual, decisive, or wise, for example, our children need to be exposed to all of these valuable traits.

Dare to Dream Big

In 2007, I was fortunate enough to visit South Africa. I have a close friend, Brennan, who played professional rugby in South Africa and he has a vision for helping orphans there by creating a bicycle ride similar to the MS-150 or the Tour de Cure. What makes this idea seem so doable is that the largest bike race in the world is held in Cape Town, South Africa each year. Once the race is over, there is virtually a pool of cyclists from all over the world who would likely love to ride for a good cause.

So we went to Cape Town to do the Cape Argus race and to film at an orphanage run by friends of Brennan from his rugby days. We hoped to raise interest and awareness back home in the states. It is, in part, because of that trip that I am committed to donating a portion of every sale of Exercising Values to ministries that help orphans there and throughout the world.

Even being a mom to six children did not prepare me for the rush of emotion I felt when little orphan children would throw their arms around me and I would realize they had no mother or father to guide and protect them. Good people are doing what they can there but the sheer volume of need is overwhelming. My vision for Exercising Values is that by helping parents give to their own children; we can also give to children who have no parents. As a customer of Exercising Values, you have already had a part in realizing that dream.

The following words written by Marianne Williamson are believed by many to have been quoted in an important speech by South Africa's greatest hero,

Nelson Mandela. I think these words speak to our desire to inspire our children to great character;

"Our deepest fear is not that we are inadequate.
Our deepest fear is that we are
Powerful beyond measure.
It is our Light, not our
Darkness, that most frightens us.
We ask ourselves, Who am I to be brilliant,
Gorgeous, talented, fabulous?
Actually, who are you not to be?
You are a child of God.
Your playing small does not serve the World.
There is nothing enlightening about
Shrinking so that other people
Won't feel unsure around you.
We were born to make manifest the
Glory of God that is within us.
It is not just in some of us; it is in everyone.
As we let our own Light shine,
We unconsciously give other people
Permission to do the same.
As we are liberated from our own fear,
Our presence automatically

Liberates others."

Help your children dream a big dream and then realize it. Use your physical fitness to help someone. It doesn't have to be on a grand scale. Just go rake the neighbor lady's leaves or shovel her driveway or mow her lawn.

Call on your own dreams to make a change in your family's health. Don't settle for post-pregnancy pounds or middle age spread. Choose to take action to ensure your own health and that of your children.

It is not narcissistic to preserve your health and appearance. In fact, is anyone inspired or benefitted by you letting yourself go? You'll have more energy and feel less stressed when you make physical fitness a daily priority.

I have one more story from South Africa for you to ponder. When 1984 Nobel Peace Prize winner, Desmond Tutu, was a child growing up under Apartheid, he witnessed his first act of respect and kindness from a white man when an Anglican priest tipped his hat as he passed Tutu's mother. Tutu later credited this expression of courtesy as a turning point in his life that caused him to have an interest in Christianity and to later become the archbishop of South Africa. He was destined to play a key role in ending Apartheid.

The character we teach our children to have may have far-reaching effects. It will open doors for them and be helpful to others. Never underestimate the power of what you are doing as you teach and encourage your children each day.

Think of the time and money people spend trying to lose weight. Free yourself and your children from this by instilling a life style of fitness. Give them the timeless gift of a sound mind in a sound body. This will free them to focus their energies on other things, to dream big dreams and to succeed.

The Need to Control Television

One of the insidious competitors for shaping your children's values is the media and television in particular. When I was a student at Stanford University oh so many years ago, I wrote a paper for a broadcast communications class on violence on television. I remember it because it was one of the first papers I wrote while there as a transfer student. I wondered how I would do in this new environment.

The professor gave me an A- and wrote that the minus came because I didn't actually solve the problem. Solve the problem? They expected me to actually solve a major social problem?

That was the first inkling I had that I was in school to actually impact the world. Truly I was flabbergasted that anyone expected me to solve a problem of such magnitude. Sadly, I never did and neither did you and we all know television has only grown more violent and more explicit since then.

My son, Skyler, commented one day that one of the reasons he enjoyed the children in Taiwan, where he visited, was they were not in his words "tainted by television." He thought they were happier and more teachable and enthusiastic. I had just read a study that just having the television on in the background will cause young children to be less active. It distracts them and actually saps their natural energy. So even if the content itself isn't a problem; it can still be detrimental to children to have the television on.

One of my personal training clients told me that when her young child was asked what his parents did he responded by saying "they kill people". Naturally she and her husband were called in to speak to school officials. Their son knew that both parents were police officers. Although neither had ever killed anyone, their son assumed from what he had seen on television, that if they were police officers, they killed people. It makes you wonder what assumptions your children might be making about how the world works because of what they've seen on television.

Shutting off the television and spending just a few minutes each day with Exercising Values will ensure that your children learn healthy fitness activities along with a character quality. Interacting with you each day will help them learn what you value most. It will help keep them from being tainted by television and the 101 other damaging influences vying for their attention. Instead, they will have a childhood full of happy memories with you.

CHAPTER FOUR
ENHANCING FAMILY LIFE THROUGH FITNESS AND TIME TOGETHER

Exercising Values assures you that every day you will be building health, fitness, and good character into your children's lives. They can count on your attention every day. By prioritizing this for even fifteen minutes a day, you are sending them the message that health is important, that character is important, but most of all, that they are important to you.

Bedtime Stories with a Purpose

Included in each day's exercise lesson are some practical tips for improving family life, some special tips just for moms, and don't forget the delightful bedtime story taken from the best in children's literature. Great literature is deemed great, in part, because it illuminates some universal truth often involving the consequences of practicing or not practicing good character.

I wanted to make it simple for you to identify some of the best stories for exploring character and to be able to relax and listen with your children while they are read. They will not only hold your children's attention; they will improve their attention span and create a love of reading. My husband, Doug, is the voice on the recordings of Tom Sawyer, Pollyanna, and all the great stories in the collection we make available to you on our website www.exercisingvalues.com

My hope is that your children will come to anticipate these fun activities that they share with you each day. They will open doors for communication with them. I hope that these meaningful moments will also bring you much happiness. I am confident that you will always consider the time you devote to this program as time well spent.

Finding Time by Staying Focused

It is so important to figure out how to spend our time. People are more important than projects but sometimes our projects are the way we support our families. In business you get paid for what you get done but with your family you get rewarded for doing, for being there. The key is keeping what's essential in both projects and relationships and tossing out the time wasters in both. If someone wastes your money, they are also wasting your time because at some point you traded your time for that money.

You are investing time and effort each day to nudge your children in the right direction. I know you want to focus and finish. If you take on too many projects, none of them may get done.

Moms are great at multi-tasking. Their ability to switch from right brain to left brain helps them tremendously to handle a lot of diverse responsibilities. But for this brief fifteen minutes let this be all you are trying to do. Turn off anything that distracts you including the phone, computer, television and radio. Clear your mind of inner distractions and let your children know you are completely there with them.

Not everything you do can be wrapped up and finished. Children are a work of art that you contribute to a little each day. In the end, they will be the best work of your life. Don't let projects distract you from this daily interaction with your children. Don't let them steal your time, money, and life away. Do a reasonable amount of the things that draw and interest you. Keep it to the ones you can actually focus on and finish, while preserving time for the people you love.

I worked hard this week and got some things done. I also took my grandson for a walk and played some game we invented that had elements of soccer, track, and gymnastics. Sometimes getting things done is over-rated especially if it means missing happy, irreplaceable moments.

Don't do it. Enjoy your moments of happiness. Exercising Values gives you a plan for how you won't miss the important things no matter how busy you are building financial support under the people you love or otherwise contributing your gifts to the world.

Life is precious and worth reflecting on. We don't want to be so busy that we have no idea if what we are busy with is truly worthwhile. Consider your dreams and desires. Henry Scougal wrote a book in 1677 called "The Life of God in the Soul of Man". In it he remarks that "The worth and excellency of a soul is to be measured by the object of it's love."

Certainly you love your family and want to give them all you can. What else are you passionate about? What else do you truly love? What are you uniquely designed to contribute to your children, your spouse, your friends, and the world? Parenting involves sacrifice but never personhood annihilation. The gift of your authentic, rested, and happy self is of immeasurable value to your family and taking some time to align your purpose to your day to day life will ensure this gift will be given.

Another author that challenges me to reflect on life is Oswald Chambers. His book, My Utmost for His

Highest, is one of my favorites. I even like the word utmost. It implies draining every bit of energy you have for a worthy goal. In our society many, many people are draining every bit of their energy; but for what? Underneath our too full lives lies the vague awareness that the hour glass is emptying.

We begin to second guess our choices unless we've taken the time to reflect on where they are taking us. I really appreciate these words that Chambers wrote: "The people who influence us the most are not those who detain us with their continual talk, but those who live their lives like the stars in the sky and 'the lilies of the field'-simply and unaffectedly. Those are the lives that mold and shape us".

We all aspire to be good influences in our children's lives and sometimes we'll give up a habit or pleasure to be that good example. Their well-being often motivates us more than our own. So here's hoping we both spend our day doing something worthwhile, something that serves others, something that we truly enjoy, and something that will have eternal value. Failing that, here's hoping at least one person's life is better today because we share the planet with them. Here's hoping that maybe that person is your child and mine.

CHAPTER FIVE
CHILD DEVELOPMENT AND THE UNIQUENESS OF EACH CHILD

Bringing out the best in children is both a privilege and a challenge. The value of the investment you are making by daily setting aside time to encourage your children cannot be over-estimated. At the very least, you are creating some great family memories.

You may also be creating lifelong habits of health and good decision making. Decisions are influenced by character and all of our lives are different because of the decisions we make. So I hope you are feeling good about adopting a plan to help you get results. You are on a journey and together we will find new ways to help you prioritize your children's well-being on a daily basis.

Exercise and Child Development

Here are a few research based observations about children that will help you understand how children respond to exercise. Both boys and girls will improve on a range of physical tests up to around age 18. Children grow at different rates with the greatest growth occurring in the first two years. This is when they will reach half of their adult height. Then growth slows until it once again accelerates at 10-12 years old for girls and 12-14 for boys. During the years between these two spurts, parents should keep physical activity fun, while concentrating on skills and lavishing their children with encouragement. The most important thing is to instill a love of movement and fitness.

Allow children and yourself to progress gradually with the workouts. Praise participation and effort. Realize that time alone will bring improvements in strength as children grow bigger and stronger. This growth lasts until age 18-20 in boys and until about 14-16 in girls. There are physical reasons for imperfect coordination before puberty that has to do with the incomplete myelination of the nerve fibers, undeveloped muscle recruitment skills, and limited ability to recruit more motor units, to name a few inhibiting factors.

All this to say, be patient if they don't naturally gravitate to good form on a complex movement such as a push-up. Encourage good form, certainly, but don't over-react if their rear end is high in the air, their hands are in front of their heads, and their shoulders are rounded. Keep modeling good form and talking about it and they will get it. When all the stabilizing muscles are developed and become coordinated with the prime movers, suddenly their back will be straight and their pelvis and shoulders will be stable. They will press up and go down with the perfect form you showed them.

So expect children to be children and not miniature adults. Don't push them and don't allow them to push themselves too hard. Children do not have the same fatigue mechanisms adults have and they tend to overheat sooner than adults. Keep an eye on them and encourage them to rest if they seem overly hot or fatigued. It should always be challenging but doable for everyone.

There will be differences in each child's abilities. The average six year old, whether boy or girl, can do five push-ups before stopping. The average twelve year old boy can do fifteen, three more that the average twelve year old girl. At eighteen, this boy will be doing twenty-five on average and the girl will still be doing twelve. At eighteen, girls have 50% of the upper body muscle mass of boys and 70% of the lower body muscle. In terms of strength relative to muscle mass, they have equal strength.

Children will enjoy improving in strength, speed, coordination, agility, and sport specific skills, especially in a positive environment. Make it your aim to let your child work from success. Build on what they can already do. Let them experience the sheer joy of movement. Practicing the raw skills of jumping, kicking, and throwing now, will help lay a foundation for more technical, sport-related skills later.

No child enjoys not feeling competent at what he does and daily practice will breed confidence and competence. Never underestimate the value of introducing exercise as a family activity. Research shows that health is enhanced by strong ties to family. The very fact that you set a special time aside each day to do this with your children sends them a message that they are loved and cared for.

If your child is a bit heavier than you wish, take heart in knowing that children are naturally good fat-burners. Their bodies prefer fat as fuel. So this consistent increase in activity will soon show in their smaller waistline. Success breeds success and they will feel better and want to move even more. There is no need to focus attention on their need to lose weight. Get them to love activity and it will come off in no time with their self-esteem intact.

Some research suggests that the moderate to high intensity intervals we do in Exercising Values represent the best way to lose body fat. Further, research also shows that intervals along with moderate length but high intensity continuous efforts are the best methods to improve endurance performance in children up until puberty. Long bouts of slower endurance work are not as suitable for children psychologically or physically and are just not necessary. Leave them wanting more.

The Exercising Values program takes into consideration how adults and children working out side by side differ. Children's heart rates may reach anaerobic threshold or even higher during interval work. In children, aerobic threshold is higher than adults who reach it at about 75% of their maximum heart rate. For children, this is more likely to be 85% of maximum heart rate and of course their maximum heart rates are naturally higher than an adult's.

When intensity, volume, frequency and duration are sufficient, young children can improve significantly in strength. Relatively, this will be the same as an adult who is training. So don't challenge them to a push-up contest unless you are prepared to lose.

Unlike adults, this improvement will not be from hypertrophy, (the increase in muscle size), and neuromuscular improvement so much as from improvements in the neuromuscular system alone. In other words, their body figures out how to recruit more of the muscle fibers they already have. So no need to fear your child will become insanely muscular with this training. It just won't happen.

This also means that the work you are doing with them today will greatly increase their athletic potential tomorrow. Before puberty, it is most appropriate to focus on coordination and stability. Learning the basic moves in the Exercising Values program and practicing them while still at a young age is a huge advantage.

They will be ready to use the good techniques they are learning now, to safely and effectively perform high intensity training when they get older. They will have developed their stabilizing muscles. Help them to pay attention to good posture and body alignment now and everything will be easier for them later.

Strength training in young children will thicken their bones by promoting increased muscle density that pulls on the bones. Just using body weight protects their growth plates, enhances their body awareness, and keeps them safe. It will also enhance their self-esteem as they witness their own improvement and as you acknowledge and praise them.

Challenging but brief exercise sessions keep them interested without pushing them to do too much. In short, the workouts in Exercising Values are ideally suited for children and will play to their strengths as well as help them overcome their weaknesses. With this strong foundation, they will be prepared to do well at any sport they later try.

Respecting Various Learning Styles

You will notice that from week to week Exercising Values will vary the way ideas are presented and will review ideas already presented. This is done deliberately in order to optimize the learning environment for every child. Learning theory originated by Howard Gardner explains what we have all observed. People perceive and understand the world around them through different pathways. The seven pathways Gardner identifies are probably not exhaustive but they will help us connect with most children by respecting their learning styles. These seven are:

Linguistic: Learning via the spoken or written word encompasses both the visual and auditory learner and will be a vital part of our program as we define and discuss the character qualities and listen to the illustrative stories.

Logical-Mathematical: This goes beyond just the ability to use numbers but also includes inductive and deductive reasoning and the ability to recognize abstract patterns. This comes into play when we decide how we will begin to display the character quality in our lives.

Visual-Spatial: Those strong in this learning style are easily able to ascertain spatial dimensions and visualize things. This will be practiced as we take the descriptions of the exercises and turn them into action first by seeing them in our minds

Body-Kinesthetic: This is a skill we are obviously emphasizing in our program as we learn to move our bodies and develop proprioception which is the sense of our body in space.

Musical-Rhythmic: We will vary the rhythm of the exercises by changing how quickly or slowly we go through each movement; sometimes exploding through a movement, sometimes going ultra slowly and sometimes using a static contraction.

Interpersonal: Surely this is at the heart of what we are doing. Working together as a family builds relationships and develops communication skills.

Intra-personal: Reflecting on the various character qualities will bring a lot of self-awareness. We will better understand our motivations and our emotions as well as the way we come across to other people.

This information makes us realize that other people including our own flesh and blood may not process information in the same way we do. Whereas one person can just listen and do; another might need you to draw a picture. In thirty years of marriage, my husband still likes to draw me pictures to explain directions.. They usually look like scratches with no meaning to me, an auditory learner. And yes, if I find something interesting, I love to read it aloud to him even though I know full well he'd rather I just hand it over so he can see it for himself. Sigh. Like everything else, incorporating these ideas into how you treat people is a process.

Knowing this, maybe we should all give classroom teachers, who inevitably deal with various learning styles every day, a deserved pat on the back for their efforts to help every student understand. In my many years of home educating my children, I recall having to work to balance the learning styles of just six or fewer learners. While doing Exercising Values some of these differences in your own children will become apparent.

One of my daughters learned math by jumping on a number line sprawled across the floor. She was always in motion and got bored when she wasn't moving. Today, she coaches gymnastics. While she could barely sit still, her older sister could sit for hours reading and today is one of the best read people I know. My oldest son could examine a patch of ground for hours, quietly observing the insects and flowers. He felt rushed if you took less than four hours at a museum. Today he is a graphic artist and a musician and is just more patient and thoughtful than most people you'll meet. Learning styles are a big part of who we are and need to be noted and appreciated.

Here's just a few more ways that people differ that you may want to consider when implementing this program. Everyone has a time of day when they are more productive, alert, and engaged. If someone is resisting the program it may turn around if you move the session from first thing in the morning to late morning, afternoon, or evening. Try not to be too set on your own personal preference. Rotating the time of day is another option.

Some people will love the group interaction and others may want to practice a new skill on their own. Some like music in the background and others just find it distracting. Be flexible on these details but also use it as a chance to teach your children about individual preferences that are neither right nor wrong, just different. Being made aware of this early in life will give them a distinct advantage in understanding and getting along with others.

Be certain that you are also easy to get long with. We can all think of times we had to spend time with people who were jaded, cynical or negative in some way. Negative or bored people are just hard to be around. On the other hand, enthusiastic, accepting people can make our day. Choose your attitude before you gather the family for Exercising Values and soon you'll be choosing to be more upbeat all day long.

At those times when you feel drained and you just can't shake the blues, try to take some time to rest and nurture yourself. Have fun or do nothing but take a break when you are about to break. The normal routine can wait, even Exercising Values.

Enhancing Learning through Labeling Good Behavior

Bandura's Social Learning Theory offers a few additional observations about the way people learn.

His first principle explores the fact that observational learning is enhanced by associating labels. So although your children may have observed you being enthusiastic, loyal, hospitable or diligent; your fine example is much more likely to be copied when it is identified and given a name. This should encourage us that when we are following the Exercising Values program; we will be evoking lasting benefits.

As you explain the benefits of practicing each character quality, your children will adopt them partly due to the admired status you naturally hold as a parent and partly because you are enabling them to understand its functional value. So just by identifying and defining a character quality that you admire, you increase the likelihood that your children will adopt that desirable trait.

What they focus on and talk about will change because "the mouth speaks what the heart is full of". Fill your child's heart with wisdom. "Whatever is true, whatever is noble, whatever is right, whatever is pure, whatever is lovely, whatever is admirable, if anything is excellent or praiseworthy let your mind think on such things. " (Philippians 4:8)

CHAPTER SIX
OVERCOMING OBSTACLES

I am always intrigued by people who say they benefit from sayings like "nothing tastes as good as skinny feels". If putting down that bagel made us instantaneously skinny, I suppose we would always choose to do so. The problem lies in that the comfort we are seeking from the bagel is right now and skinny will be many foregone bagels later if at all. It all comes down to delayed gratification. Are you willing to give up momentary pleasure or comfort and have faith that by doing so you will gain greater pleasure and comfort down the line?

I'm also disturbed when I hear people being dismissive about slow metabolisms, thyroid issues, genetic factors, hormonal issues, gender differences, age-related hinderances, busy lifestyles, stress or any of the other reasons people give for why it is hard for them to lose weight. I remember an old sitcom episode where a pregnant woman goes to the hospital with Braxton Hicks contractions and when her male friend acts dismissive because it was just false labor pains she cuts him off with,"No uterus. No opinion." I think that sums it up. So rather than dismiss those things someone else feels overwhelmed by in their struggle to lose weight; I think it makes more sense to acknowledge that they are real hinderances that need to be overcome.

Maybe you weren't given the easiest body to work with and maybe your child is struggling with the same genes. Recently a study from the University of Florida tied childhood ear infections to adult obesity. We may never know all the reasons why controlling weight seems to be so much harder for some than for others.

Researchers are finding weight loss is made more difficult by pollution, pesticides, exhaust fumes, plastics and a lot more. Accepting that you may have to be a little more consistent with healthy eating and exercise than someone else is the first step. Don't let it keep you from trying.

I'll never understand how Helen Keller came to have the complex vocabulary ascribed to her from her lectures, when she was unable to see or hear. We're all inspired by amputees who run road races and the like. Just last week, I ran next to a man in a race who had lost a leg in Iraq. He not only runs races, he wanted to re-enlist.

Don't quit because it gets hard. If you continue with this program, you will have improved fitness and a closer family life for a long time to come. That will be your reward for your diligence now.

Developing an Action Plan

Once you have determined to overcome obstacles, the practical step of where to begin comes in. I recommend an exercise where you trace your biggest obstacle backwards until you find a first step on which you can take action. For example, you simply fill in the blank with a statement such as:

I don't enjoy the weekends because:

_____.

Let's say you answered "because we always just stay home".

Then you would say:

We always stay home because:

_____.

"we can't think of anything fun to do"

We can't think of anything fun to do because

_____.

"we never talk about it"

We never talk about it because

_____.

"we never think to do so"

Aha, you are thinking about it now; so a first step would be to get the family together to talk about what would be fun to do this weekend. This exercise will help you to find some action you can take toward any goal you have, like enjoying your weekends more. Then work backwards until that big obstacle tumbles. What you are doing is important so it is worth the time to overcome obstacles.

Your Call to Action

The culture is going the wrong way and like a moving stream our children are being caught up in it while we sometimes stand helplessly by. The first time I went white water rafting the man in front of me grabbed me as the raft threw him into the icy cold water. I used all the strength I had trying to avoid it but soon found myself on alert thrashing in the water. At first, the raft actually bounced over and on top of me. When it became clear to me that no one on the raft was going to rescue me, I spotted a rock and swam to it.

It was very cold, there was a sensation of being pulled down, and my mind turned to a friend who had drowned in a lake. I was calm but I knew I couldn't survive on that rock for long so I sprinted to the next raft. At orientation, they had taught us to allow the person in the raft to dunk us under to help get the momentum to pull us into the raft. I believed that I was so drained at that point that if for any reason they failed to pull me in after dunking me under that I would not have the strength to make it. So I insisted that they just pull me up without the push under and soon I was safely on board.

You have made a decision to try the program in this book. I implore you to try it for a full month. We can drown if we go from raft to raft looking for someone to rescue us. Get to the raft. Get what you need. Get safely on board. The danger is real and someone is offering you a hand. Please take it.

CHAPTER SEVEN
CHOOSE TO ENJOY YOUR LIFE MORE BY CONTROLLING STRESS

Stress Relief for Busy Parents

Controlling stress has many benefits both now and as an investment in our future. Stress actually accelerates the rate at which cells age so controlling stress has significant anti-aging benefits. Chronic stress raises the level of insulin in the blood and raises cortisol levels which causes inflammation and thus disease.

Too much sugar is definitely a stress to the body as it will also independently raise insulin levels. When insulin is up, fat burning stops. Even blood sugar promotes fat loss. Studies show that caffeine, along with stress, also contributes to elevated cortisol levels. High cortisol levels cause fat to be preferentially stores in the abdominal area. A vicious circle is created when we feel additional stress because of the fat we are gaining because of our stress.

Some stress just can't be avoided. A recent study from the University of California looked at the effects of caring for children with chronic illness and they found that it ages the moms by as much as ten years. Only you can assess the amount of stress you are under but please take stress reduction seriously. Some daily happy moments with your children could literally turn back the clock. If you think you don't have time to commit to Exercising Values each day, it may be that you don't have enough time not to.

Stress increases the risk of obesity and promotes inter-abdominal fat. It raises cholesterol over time and even accelerates inflammatory gum disease which in turn promotes heart disease. Even happy events such as a move, a vacation, or exercise contribute to the stress load. Not all stress can or should be avoided but unnecessary harmful stress should certainly be addressed. We all need to learn how to take a break.

Remember health and character are intertwined. The effort you are making to teach character has the added health benefit of protecting the body from stress and therefore acidity. Studies have shown that anger, unforgivingness, and bitterness in particular put the body in a stressed and acidic mode.

Staying calm and breathing deeply provides more oxygen to the cells and this in turn fights disease. Faith and prayer are health promoting. In the Bible Gods says "I know the plans I have for you, plans to help and not to harm you; to give you a hope and a future." Trust Him as you seek to practice good character and to pass it on to your children.

I want to give you several more suggestions for reducing stress. The entire Exercising Values program is, of course, a main defense against stress. When you know you are daily investing in the people who are most important to you, you will feel less trapped by the daily grind and time wasters. Stress is something we can alleviate. With the right daily routine that includes laughter, exercise, wholesome foods, sleep, friends, and relaxation we can find a brighter, happier and healthier future.

Ten tips to reduce stress

1. Work From a List (or don't)
Sometimes we feel stressed simply because we have this vague feeling that we are not attending to urgent or important matters. Management experts often recommend keeping a current list of on-going projects that you can review at least once a week. They insist this will lead to stress-free productivity. Maybe you should listen to them.

I believe lists like that suit some personality types and torture others. Then there will be some who immediately misplace the list and then stress and worry about that. If you like lists, you probably already have one. If you don't, try it but don't feel like a failure if it doesn't work for you.

Some people just don't function that way. However, keep in mind that one or more of your children may love the structure and accountability of lists so by all means teach them this skill. You can certainly make a list out of the Exercising Values workouts and they may love keeping a record of their achievement.

2. Exercise

When tempted to skip the daily Exercising Values routine remember that the right form of exercise will not only strengthen our bones and muscles; it will also relieve stress. It will restore emotional balance and enhance harmony between mind and body. Many find participation in sports to be particularly relaxing and enjoyable. Others feel the same way about Pilates, yoga, or taking a walk.

Exercise improves cognitive function so it's beneficial to do before school. Home schooled students who use Exercising Values as part of their physical education will find studying easier. Progressive public schools have found great gains in restoring endurance and fitness promoting exercise to their curriculum.

3. Affection and Sex

A robust sex life enhances confidence as well as health. It improves your appearance, your sleep, and your energy. One study involving 3,500 participants found that the strongest correlation to a youthful appearance is an active sex life. It can increase fitness, decrease depression, increase self-esteem, enhance intimacy, and improve the overall quality of life. It's a strong motivator for taking care of yourself, in general.

Young parents put so much focus on their children and they're tired so they can forget to be crazy in love. Don't do that. Sneak off and do something outrageous together or enjoy a quiet moment at home if that's more your style.

To suit both of you, you may need to do both. That give and take enlivens your life because you are trying to get along with and please someone who is so different from you. In the process, you become a richer, deeper person.

Sex is visual. There I've said it but surely you've noticed it, too. Many busy moms will let their appearance and fitness level slide in an effort to take care of everyone else. In the end, this benefits no one. Your marriage has a life of its own apart from the family life you enjoy with your children.

With a little creativity, you can take care of yourself and enjoy your marriage while still providing for your children. Taking time each day to do a program that builds health and admirable character for your children will keep you more relaxed so you can enjoy the rest of your life.

To truly influence our children toward health and well-being they need to see us practicing solid health habits like exercise and not just asking them to do so. Your radiant health and happiness will inspire them and be a gift to your spouse as well.

Taking care of yourself is an important part of taking care of your family. Rather than taking anything away from your children, when you do this program they get a wonderful physical education program while you get leaner and less stressed. You'll be able to channel this energy back into your marriage and everyone will be happier.

After years of personal training, I've observed that people decide when they will age. If they think of themselves as old at thirty they become old at thirty and if they think of themselves as young at sixty or seventy they project youth and give off wonderful energy. You can't fake this. It is what it is.

What you choose to do by way of new people and new experiences will impact how you see yourself. I recently saw a man and a woman receive a standing ovation from a room full of athletes after they each won their age group at a national triathlon competition. They are both eighty-five years old.

4. Eliminate Clutter
I used to clutter my house with books on how to de-clutter my house. If you share this problem, borrow a saying from Nike and just do it. Seriously, it took a move after twenty-six years in the same house raising six children to finally force the issue. You can't image

how great it is to own less stuff. That's one reason why Exercising Values requires no equipment.

Let's make a deal. Follow-up books to Exercising Values may include bands, the exercise ball, TRX, or my personal favorite for families The Lebert Buddy System. Make a deal with yourself right now that you won't let yourself buy any of that equipment unless your clutter problem has been solved. Believe me, no one is more sympathetic about why you have this problem but no one could urge you more to address it.

5. Visualize Success
It's stressful to have no idea what you are trying to accomplish with your life or in your children's lives. Purpose dispels stress. Take time to define what success is to you and then go for it.

Take 5-15 minutes when you won't be disturbed by people or phone calls. Get comfortable and fully relax. Begin to think about what you will look like and how you will feel when you have been consistently following the Exercising Values program.

See the physical and the internal changes in your mind. Picture living with people who are devoted to developing good character and a healthy body. See yourself as an important part of this family commitment. Be specific.

Review this image at least three times each day. First thing in he morning and just before sleep would be two good times to make this part of your daily routine. Or do it while brushing your teeth or while taking a shower. Changing your body, improving your family life and carving a little more time for what you believe is most important all begins in your mind. Don't limit yourself. Improve your thoughts and you'll improve your life.

6. Give Someone a Hug
Don't let this purpose driven activity become so serious that you forget to practice simple acts of affection like a pat on the back or a hug. Research abounds that children and adults need demonstrations of affection. Research aside, take a moment to completely relax and let your mind drift to

a time as a child when someone held you, or touched you and made you feel better. Then think of how that made you feel.

Now let your mind go to some time as an adult when you had a similar experience. Enjoy the memory and then go to a time when you needed to be hugged or touched but it was withheld from you. All these years later, you still remember. There's your insight. Whether a study says we need six or seven positive touches a day, we all know we really can't give or get too many. The quality of life depends on it.

7. Practice Positive Self-Talk

"As a man thinks in his heart so is he." (Proverbs 3:27) One study, (Crum et all, 2007), showed that this Biblical principle applies to weight loss and fitness. Eight-four women who were cleaning hotel rooms for a living were divided into two groups. One served as the control group. The other was told (falsely) that their occupation fulfilled the Surgeon General's standard for an active life.

Behaviors did not change between the two groups but the latter were given examples of how their work was the equivalent to significant exercise. These women began to believe that they were now athletic. Their bodies responded by losing weight, lowering body fat, lowering blood pressure, and decreasing their body mass index and waist to hip ratio!

Again, no change in actual behavior had occurred. So shall we just think ourselves thin, strong, fast? Try it and see. My recommendation is simply to recognize that your thoughts are a critical element to your success or failure. Amazing results may just be a few thoughts away.

A medical doctor recently shared with me that the brain is particularly receptive to "why" questions. If you want to lose weight, you say to yourself, "why do I always eat light and healthy food?" She explained that the brain tries to answer the question and the net result is you will begin to prefer eating light and healthy food. If you have struggled with getting results from visualization or positive affirmations in the past, this tool may offer you better results. You can use it for anything. Why do I always get plenty of sleep? Why am I such an enthusiastic person? You'll never know if this will work for you unless you try it.

It might be a good idea to inventory the thoughts you have about your athletic or weight loss goals. I don't expect you to jot down every one of your 50,000-100,000 daily thoughts but do try to note recurring themes such as "I'll never lose weight", "my entire family is overweight" or "I'm too slow, too old, too lazy to ever get results." Also, note upbeat self-messages like "that was a great workout, I am really on track" or I'm getting healthier and I feel so good!" You probably already know which type of self-talk you are experiencing. You just may not realize how much it is impacting your results.

Negative self-talk produces momentary stress relief by making it seem that there is nothing to be done. It's just an excuse, really. In the long run, it will hamper performance. It is not unlike the dieter who eats a chocolate bar for the temporary happiness it brings even though the consequences of repeatedly doing so is the antithesis of what will help her reach her weight-loss goals.

Owning up to the fact that you are getting something by being negative will actually help you change the habit. It feels good to have an excuse. It feels better to succeed.

I'm counting on you to avoid futility and hopelessness in your thoughts. Remember the Biblical principle to "do everything without complaining or arguing." Choose to believe that as you apply sound fitness principles that they will work for you. Trying to improve is stressful and this stress won't disappear. But you will be better equipped to handle it when you give a little thought to your thoughts. Try to say something positive to yourself right now.

8. Pray
Turn all your cares over to God because He cares for you. "Be anxious for nothing but in everything with prayer and supplication let your requests be made known unto God and the peace of God which passes understanding will keep your hearts in Christ

Jesus." (Philippians 4:6) Seeking God's help should always be our first resort. The fruit of the spirit is love, joy, peace, patience, kindness, goodness, faithfulness, gentleness and self-control. (Galatians 5:22-23) God is the example of all good character and the source of hope and love. He is the one who equips us to handle whatever happens in life.

9. Become Part of a Group

Despite my trip into the water, I loved my first day of white water rafting. I felt energized by the knowledge that we had to work together to stay upright and we had to be ready to rescue each other if we fell in. Is there a better analogy for what we parents need to do for each other? If you are a single parent, I hope you have a reliable friend who will support and encourage you and rescue you when needed.

We need to hold to a standard, to stand in the gap, to put a finger in the dyke. Commit to the fight to preserve a compass and a code for your children. We can try to do it alone but joining a community is a huge advantage. There are neighborhood play groups, church groups, and organizations like

M.O.P.S. The online interactive Exercising Values community is another way to stay connected to people who share your commitment. You may become the one who is pulling someone who is struggling into the boat.

10. Set Aside Time for What's Important

It is the heart of the Exercising Values program to reflect on what's important and to set aside time to devote to it. Feel very good about your choice to do this. Don't stop there. As you begin to see the value of consistent action taken over a period of time, let it inspire you to schedule time for your other goals. It may be time to read or study, a date night, or even to get a little more sleep if you need it.

CHAPTER EIGHT
TAKE RESPONSIBILITY FOR YOUR CURRENT PHYSICAL FITNESS

Are you blaming anyone else for your weight or for being out of shape? I taught two fitness classes in the early AM on the day I'm writing this. As I'm shuffling myself from a cycle class to a yoga class, it begins to pour. At that moment, I notice that my seat belt isn't fastened and as always I think of my mother who didn't believe in seat belts and refused to wear them; during my impressionable years, no less.

Yes, my mom has been dead for over ten years now but when I neglect my own safety there is a part of my mind that is blaming my mother. Then I sigh because I am a mother and I wonder what I'll be on the hook for years from now.

It's not rational or charitable to blame her, I realize, but there it is. She had a fear that she'd be trapped in a car after an accident and be unable to get her seat belt open. She was also part of that last generation where it was more common for women not to drive and she never did. During the car pool years when my sister, who also has six children, and I would get together and commiserate about our packed schedules, we wondered if instead of being a coward maybe mom was a genius.

Is anything more unproductive than blame? I compete in triathlons. Sometimes I catch the blame for a potential bad race spinning around in the back of my mind. Nothing compelling, just the usual list of work, injuries, global warming… you know. The list is on standby just in case. In every rational moment, of course, I know I am solely responsible for the outcome of that race just like I am responsible for remembering to fasten my seat belt.

Maybe it's best to not even acknowledge those half formed thoughts that we'd never speak out loud. But I suspect they affect us more than we'll ever know. So for today, I'll fasten that seat belt, prepare for my races, think fondly of my mother, and try not to give my own children too much material for the back of their minds. By the way, they do all wear their seat belts so there's hope their children won't place any blame at all. But I doubt it.

Finding Fitness Friendly Food

We are responsible for what we eat. To think otherwise is to invite weight gain. Support your exercising body with good nutrition. A lifestyle change that involves gradual healthy changes to your diet and consistent daily activity will give you many rewards. So enjoy yourself along the way and don't over-monitor your results and fret if they don't seem to be coming quickly enough. When you drink water instead of soda, cut out fried foods and fast foods, eat more fruits and vegetables, cut out processed grains, and reduce sweets; you will look and feel better.

The American Journal of Clinical Nutrition once published a series of recommendations from nutritionists around the world. The consensus was that the healthiest diet includes vegetables, whole grains, fruits, and beans. It may include some fish a few times a week but generally avoids a lot of meat and refined grains.

We can both continue to read what the research reveals and I'll be sharing these findings regularly on my blog along with my recommendations. Balance that with your own common sense. The information in this book is certainly not intended as medical advice but rather as a reminder to act on what you know and to discuss diet with your doctor or health care practitioner. New research is constantly becoming available and it is a good idea to stay on top of it. I'm committed to helping you do that.

I am not an expert on cancer research but some interesting information has crossed my desk recently which you may want to discuss with your medical doctor or research on your own. Some researchers believe that an effective way to battle cancer is to starve the cancer cells by not feeding them certain foods, such as sugar and acid forming meats.

One theory is that eating less meat may free the body to use enzymes to attack cancer cells rather than being diverted to digestion. On the other hand, a diet of fresh vegetables and juices, whole grains, nuts, seeds, and fruits will create an alkaline environment that stifles cancer. Cancer may also feed on mucus. For many people dairy products and wheat products cause mucus. This may be another reason to avoid foods to which you are sensitive or allergic.

Realize that there is a health cost when you ingest pesticides and fungicides and a benefit to avoiding them. Most people eat less when eating organic foods. Maybe this is because the nutrients shut down cravings or the superior taste is more satisfying or perhaps it is due to what you are not ingesting. In any case, fat loss will likely be the result of replacing mass-produced foods with organic, fresh food.

Selecting healthy foods means considering how they were grown and shipped. With few exceptions, our bodies cannot manufacture the vitamins and minerals they need and must get them from plants that have absorbed minerals from the soil. Poor soil, therefore, means poor food values. Shipping and storage can also compromise food values. Thus, it is best to buy local, organic produce that has been vine or tree-ripened whenever possible.

You may also want to back up your careful food choices with a high quality multi-vitamin and mineral supplement. However, no vitamin pill should be relied upon to compensate for a poor diet. I would always say food first. Your health care provider can advise. Always check with your primary healthcare professional before taking any new supplement. Some nutritional supplements can be contraindicated for people with certain health conditions.

Nutrition for bone health is a concern for women especially those who have nursed babies. The ability to convert sunshine to Vitamin D diminishes with age and can be thwarted by sunscreen. Care to ingest calcium rich foods and get a little sunshine will go a long way to offer protection from osteoporosis. More than 8 million American women have osteoporosis, a disorder characterized by porous, fragile bones.

Another 34 million Americans have its precursor, osteopenia, or diminished bone mass.

A daily multi-vitamin and mineral supplement that includes calcium, K2, boron, silicon, and magnesium will help to prevent bone loss and recent evidence says they may also help stimulate new bone growth. There is a considerable body of evidence that certain supplements can fight the damaging effects of stress. These include Vitamin C, Omega 3 fish oil, Ginseng, Gogi juice, Alpha Lipoic acid, and Gingko Biloba among others.

Consider drinking a glass of water possibly with lemon first thing in the morning. Drink water before you feel thirsty during exercise and let your thirst guide you after the workout and throughout the day. The sooner children learn that water is the go to drink when thirsty the better. Squeeze a little orange into it occasionally to make it special. It's best to get a water filter for your home and to avoid drinking from plastic especially if that plastic bottle has been left in a hot car. PCB free plastic is the best plastic to use when necessary.

Soda pop has nothing to recommend it. Recently it was discovered that corn syrup has high levels of damaging mercury. Add that to the fat producing empty calories, bone demineralization, and the like and you'll see that avoiding soda and adopting a water habit is one of the best habits you can help your child establish. Most of us don't need to be convinced that water is more preferable for our health than soft drinks but knowing and doing are two different things. See if this is a change you and your children can make together.

Children aren't the only ones to benefit from drinking more water. It can be key to keeping your own weight down. Dehydration spells stress to your body and it will release hormones to fight it. Drinking more water will reduce appetite and soothe late night eating urges. It will improve performance. Add all that up and you'll see why drinking adequate amounts of water will help you reach or keep your ideal body weight. I'll drink to that!

By the way, perceiving the body's need for water lessens with age so you may be more chronically dehydrated than you realize. If you do not consume enough fresh water every day, your body will age faster, appear fatter, have less endurance, be more susceptible to illness, lose joint mobility, and much more. Generally speaking, most children require no less than 8-10 glasses per day and adults require about 12-16 glasses per day. A diet very high in fresh fruits and vegetables may reduce these numbers somewhat.

Begin each day with water to reinforce your commitment to drink it throughout the day. Providing your children with a water bottle will remind them to drink often. Stainless steel or PCB free plastic may be a safer option than regular plastic water bottles. At home, you may want to also choose glass over plastic cups.

John Hopkins Medical Center has recently issued warnings against using plastic in the microwave or freezer. This includes water bottles and plastic wrap. Dioxins in plastic have been implicated in causing cancer, especially breast cancer. High heat causes it to leach out of the plastic and on to your food. Glass, corning ware, and even a paper towel are better choices. Prevention is always preferable to treatment so don't sacrifice your long-term health for short-term convenience.

Food preparation and storage is important. Home cooking has become a lost art but one worth restoring. The University of Arkansas recently published a study showing that up to 93% of people eating in restaurants underestimate the calories they are consuming. Just eating at home will help you stay lean. But it can't be an ordeal or you won't make it a habit. That means you need to plan so you can have healthy ingredients available.

Make a large pot of soup at the beginning of the weekend and enjoy the convenience of avoiding the slow death, I mean, fast food line. When you are tired and hungry it needs to be simple so keep vegetables, fruits, lean meats, raw nuts, beans, Vega products, Ezekial bread and other similar items on hand. Eat some of your food raw and you'll feel better.

Better food choices means better health. Being drawn to foods that are antioxidant-rich and anti-inflammatory will help our families stay healthy and if needed to also burn body fat while preserving muscle mass. Here's a brief list of some of the nutritional needs that today's children sometimes lack. It will help us make improvements to guard their well-being.

Vitamin E

Two-thirds of preschoolers and 80% of U.S. kids under 8 fall short of this important vitamin. Avocado, peanut butter, and sunflower seeds are some kid-friendly sources.

Calcium and Vitamin D

Vitamin D and calcium work together to promote bone health. Nutrients work synergistically rather than in isolation. Vitamin D improves muscle strength, thereby reducing fracture risk through falls. High blood levels of vitamin D also prevent the loss of calcium from bones

Vitamin D is currently under careful scrutiny by researchers. These investigations indicate that many people may need more Vitamin D than what is currently recommended. It may be the key to preventing a host of diseases including colorectal, breast and prostate cancers, autoimmune diseases such as multiple sclerosis, as well as high blood pressure and cardiovascular diseases.

A few daily minutes of sunshine without sunscreen, between April and August will help give children the vitamin D necessary to utilize dietary calcium. Food sources are limited but include fish oil and fortified foods. Soft drinks leach minerals from bones and should be avoided.

About one-third of U.S. children ages 4-8 don't get enough calcium and this jumps to 90% for teenage girls. Dairy products, dark leafy greens, broccoli, salmon with bones, dried beans and peas, and almonds are good sources. Interestingly, olive oil has also been shown to aid bone growth in children.

Non-dairy sources of calcium are obviously preferable for people with lactose intolerance or a milk allergy. Allergies to dairy and wheat are quite common and will cause inflammation and a variety of symptoms. If you suspect food allergies in yourself or in your child you may be surprised by how much better you will feel when they are eliminated.

You may want to consult your doctor for allergy testing. These tests are simple. I had them as a child because I was always getting sick with bronchitis and pneumonia. I missed fifty days of kindergarden due to respiratory illnesses. With testing, my parents discovered that I was allergic to casein, the protein in milk, and a host of other environmental allergies. Discovering your child's sensitivities may be the first step toward feeling better.

Fiber

Though we often associate this need with adults, the truth is children need nearly as much fiber as adults with the current recommendation being 19-25 grams a day. Fiber comes from plants, not animals. Refined, processed foods have had most if not all of their fiber removed.

Good sources of fiber that children will enjoy include: hummus, whole wheat bread, berries, apples, beans, lentils, oatmeal, and sweet potatoes.

Soluble fiber binds bile acids and draws cholesterol out of the bloodstream. It slows the absorption of carbohydrates which helps keep blood sugar levels even through the next meal and it curbs appetite.

Insoluble Fiber softens your stool and increases its bulk. It also curbs appetite. It can be found in the peels and skins of fruit. Naturally occurring fiber rich foods have many additional benefits and are far superior to fiber supplements or bran cereals.

Cinnamon
Just ¼ teaspoon of cinnamon will help stabilize blood sugar for days or even weeks and can be enjoyed as a tea. Keeping blood sugar level is important to body composition. If blood sugar levels are too low, we cannot nourish our muscles and they begin to break

down. Muscle mass preserves our metabolism and our shape.

If insulin levels are too high they inhibit the body's ability to burn fat for energy so more fat is stored. Sprinkling cinnamon on oatmeal cooked from scratch is much more satisfying than settling for instant cereal laced with cinnamon sugar. You can add stevia to sweeten but may find apple slices are all the sweetener you need.

Protein
Protein builds and repairs. It promotes mental alertness. Until recently, all three of my sons chose to be vegetarians while my husband and three daughters did not. Now one son has taken up meat and two of the girls have switched to a vegetarian lifestyle.

I have chosen a vegetarian lifestyle for years at a time and at other times I have opted to eat animal proteins on the advise of my physician. Recently, my preference is to mostly eat plant sources of protein with some fish a few times a week. However, on occasion I do include a little chicken or beef.

When my oldest son first asked to be a vegetarian at age five, I confess I was nervous. Over time, I have seen him grow past six feet in perfect health. So feel free to explore the many sources of protein beyond lean meat and eggs. This includes beans, nuts, seeds, vegetables, grains, hemp and more. Eating your protein first helps suppress appetite because proteins are digested more slowly than carbohydrates, even ones with lots of fiber. If you have questions, a nutritionist can assist you.

Fish is an excellent low fat choice for protein. Research has shown that people who eat fish are less likely to suffer from heart disease and cancer. Unfortunately, some fish is tainted by mercury so we may need to limit how much we consume.

Due to the possibility of mercury contamination, it is important to check the latest information on safe levels. If mercury accumulates in the body it can harm the brain and nervous system and children and unborn babies are particularly vulnerable to its damaging effects. People with thyroid problems also need to be careful to avoid excessive mercury consumption.

Some weight loss experts recommend eating about fifteen grams of non-processed white meat turkey breast a couple hours before bed. This assists in fat loss. It also promotes sleep and growth hormone release from the tryptophan it contains. If you have trouble controlling late night snacking this might be a way to avoid empty calories while not feeling deprived. It will help you break the bad habit of stuffing yourself just before bed.

Omega-3 Rich Fish Oil or Flaxseed
Omega-3 rich foods reduce fat storage and promote the loss of existing body fat. They stabilize blood sugar levels and lower insulin levels. They decrease appetite and improve mood and energy levels. They can improve attention span. They reduce inflammation and improve the immune system. They strengthen the heart and stabilize the heart rhythm,

prevent blood clots, lower triglycerides and blood pressure, and improve the elasticity of blood vessels.

They also improve skin quality. I add that because people sometimes tune out long lists of disease prevention but tune into what will make them look better. No problem. If that's your true motivation you will still get the associated health benefits.

Potassium

You'll be eating more fruit, avocados and sweet potatoes to get this one. Bananas, oranges, pistachios, dried apricots, and cod are also good sources. Since children are only getting about 40% of what they need it's important to include these foods in their diet.

Iron

Low iron is especially common in over-weight children. A chronic deficit can cause learning and behavior problems. Meat, beans, lentils, and raisins will help raise these levels.

Enzymes

Raw foods and the enzymes they contain assist in the digestion and absorption of food. Beneficial enzymes are destroyed above 104 degrees Fahrenheit or 40 degrees Celsius so it is important to eat a large portion of your foods raw. Enzyme-rich foods include fresh fruits and vegetables, nuts, seeds, sprouted grains, and other foods that have not been processed. Refrigerate these items, including nuts and seeds, because otherwise they lose nutritional value and might even turn rancid.

Carotenoid Rich Foods

Anti-oxidant rich carotenoids may play a role in rejuvenating cells and thus they may play a role in reducing disease causing inflammation and in preserving youth. Broccoli, cauliflower, winter squash, red and yellow peppers, cantaloupe, spinach, kale, egg yolks, lobster, shrimp, and salmon all contain carotenoids.

Your choices will Influence Future Generations

The liver is a key organ for successful fat-burning. Reducing alcohol has benefitted some clients of mine who were plateauing in their weight loss. This is an area that you may benefit by consulting a physician that is knowledgeable about nutrition. I often refer clients to the doctor I personally work with and many of these clients have seen dramatic improvements in their overall health, weight loss, and energy by adopting a diet that supports the liver.

My mother and my aunt died of liver disease so I am tuned into liver health and try to avoid things that tax the liver like unnecessary over-the-counter drugs. These attitudes will be picked up by your children. Balance this, by helping them understand that there is a time and a place for certain drugs.

When my youngest daughter, Hilary, was seventeen years old she suffered a severely sprained ankle at her national basketball tournament. She had traveled with the team so I wasn't there. She was refusing the pain medication offered her at the emergency room. I had to encouraged her to take the pain medicine as soon as I heard she was refusing it.

I later learned from a MD that specializes in sports medicine that avoiding anti-inflammatories in the first 24 hours will actually speed healing so maybe there was some benefit in her delay. I hope so for all the pain she felt. It was a sobering realization to know that while in such intense pain, she was still choosing to emulate choices she had seen me make regarding pain medication.

Parenting by example occurs whether or not we are aware of our influence and it never ends. When your child grows up and is the age you are now they will recall how you lived at that age and possibly choose to copy your example. It will never be as simple as teaching them what to do. You also need to model the lifestyle you are recommending. I'm a personal trainer and I learned a long time ago that our habits get scrutinized by clients, co-workers and people in the gym who note what we eat and don't eat and how we work out. What we do influences other people's choices. They like to see that you walk the talk.

It's Okay to Fail Occasionally, Even When All Eyes Are on You

When I was nine years old one of the two elm trees in my front yard was split in two by lightning. The fallen tree provided great places to build forts and play all sorts of games. After my dad ended that by hauling all the brush away, I noticed another way to fit the tree into my playtime.

Where the tree had split there was a piece of the tree just large enough for me to slip one of my mother's Folger's coffee cans over it so I could use it as a target. I stepped back and tossed a soft ball at it. Bang, it hit the can. I'd repeat that for hours. I did this ritual off and on for a couple summers. If there was anything I knew how to do, it was toss an accurate pitch.

In college, a group of my friends joined a slow pitch league where you pitched to your own team. We needed a pitcher. Done. I was born for the job or so I thought. The first game, I promise you, every single person I knew on this earth came to watch that game. With my prior years of experience, I hadn't bothered to practice so sure I was of my ability to hit the can or throw so my team mate could hit the ball. I could not have been more wrong.

Do you have a most embarrassing moment? Well, this is one of mine. I cannot tell you what happened to me that day but I could not let go of that ball. Consequently, I pitched it straight up in the air not once but over and over again. I began to panic thinking this just can't be happening. After an excruciatingly long time, someone made me stop and another pitcher was brought in.

I tell you this to say that even when you are in your element and you have prepared and think you know what you are doing, you will at times fail. We are not going to be perfect parents. You may embarrass your kids or they may embarrass you. I know that feeling but get into the game anyway.

People on their way to doing great things will fail along the way. Thomas Edison's journey to make a light bulb is often used to illustrate this point. When asked about his many failed attempts and queried as to whether he should just quit, he said: "Why would I ever give up? I now know definitely over 9,000 ways that an electric light bulb will not work. Success is almost in my grasp." We have light because he persevered through at least an additional 1,000 attempts. You can be a light to your children if you are willing to step up and be a role model.

I think one of those balls actually landed behind me. I'm sure it was hilarious to watch. I lived to pitch another day and so will you.

CHAPTER NINE
GETTING LEAN WHILE RAISING LEAN AND HAPPY CHILDREN

If you look at the research concerning self-esteem and body composition, you'd wonder how an expression "fat and happy" ever took root. The truth is, being overweight is a common cause of depression in children. Researchers disagree as to how much of this has a physical cause and how much is caused by social pressure. However, everyone seems to agree that children feel better about themselves when they are closer to their ideal body weight.

The good news is that because they are still growing their bodies will work with them to help them lose unwanted body fat. With this program, you also become their ally in this effort without singling them out in any way.

What about you? For some women, childbearing brings with it an abandonment of responsibility for how their body looks and performs. Many women, long after their last baby is born, trace their current weight problems back to pregnancy. To solve any problem you have to take some responsibility.

You may have been busy with more important things or at least things that seemed more important at the time. There was sleep deprivation. There were lots of adjustments. You may have been so involved with the care and well-being of your baby that self-care and the well-being of your own body were seen as selfish and unimportant.

Rarely is that excuse truly the case. Staying healthy and energetic is a gift to your children. It makes you more available to them. It may prolong your life so you'll enjoy the fruits of your labor like grandchildren and special times with your grown children.

Do you want your child to grow into a healthy middle aged person free from lifestyle induced disease and free from constant weight-related health concerns? Then give them a model of how to do that. You raise your children longer than you think, longer than you'll even be alive. They will always turn over in their minds the way you did things. Choose to care about your body and your health. You don't have to be obsessed with it or give it more importance than it deserves but "keeping your body under" (1 Corinthians 9:27) is a worthy goal.

While you are helping yourself you are also providing a firm foundation for your children. By associating healthy food and activity with love and acceptance you are setting them up for a lifetime of good choices. Do you really want them to equate cookies with love? You can choose the associations they make.

Just because other people associate fun with junk food doesn't mean you have to do it. Walk down the soda aisle and feel the satisfaction of rejecting millions of advertising dollars spent to convince you that empty calories spell fun. Dress up the water or juice you serve your children with a colorful umbrella or straw. Then spend a few minutes with them and they are on their way to a lifetime of healthy water drinking. Celebrate every special occasion with soda pop and guess what your grandchildren will likely be drinking every special moment of their life.

Weight Loss 101

Let's look at how excess body fat comes to reside on our bodies. Young or old the process is basically the same. Although, there are some special concerns for moms that we will go into later. The short answer to the basic problem is that more calories have been ingested than have been burned off.

When there was a surplus of energy it was stored as fat. When we create a deficit of energy, whether it is from more activity or fewer calories, we will expend the stored energy i.e. burn body fat. It's important to recognize that this is a universal truth and if your experience contradicts it in some way then we need to do some detective work to see why it doesn't seem to be working.

Before we go any further we need to get honest. Do you really have no idea why you or your son or daughter are carrying extra pounds? For example, if you know what habitual empty calories you are eating then the next step would be to strategize to cut down or eliminate them. Complex formulas for determining caloric needs have their place but if you know you or your child are eating a bag of chips or a bowl of ice cream several nights a week; just start there and save the tweaking for later. Start with what you already know.

If making a small change like eliminating a certain snack food or dessert seems easy enough, then you are on your way. You just needed to become more aware of what you were eating. Many people will not find this that easy. When they attempt to make even the smallest change they begin to feel confined, deprived, or rebellious.

At the deepest level, they resist the very change they initiated. At root, they want to feel loved and comforted, even spoiled. Somewhere along the line these foods have grown to mean a form of love.

You need to be brutally honest and see this food not as your problem but as your solution. It is solving a longing in your heart. Consciously you may know it's not a very good solution; but there it is. You are doing the best you can to take care of yourself and so is your child. A house divided against itself will not stand and you will not win a battle against yourself; a part of you will lose.

Try this. Is there anything that you can access as easily as food when you need comfort, stimulation, or pleasure? We've all seen the lists: take a walk, drink some tea, hot bath, phone a friend, etc. This can work but often doesn't because everything on the list is harder to reach for than a cookie.

Take some time to really think of something that you want; something that makes you feel cared for and help your child to do the same. It may even be a low-calorie food that you don't allow yourself because of expense. Out of season fruit or a glass of Perrier with lime might be as much of a reward as a piece of chocolate cake if you see it as a forbidden treat.

Just try it. Even if it doesn't work for you it may be the perfect strategy for your child. Over-consumption is a complex problem and there may be many smaller changes and solutions that add up rather than one magic change that suddenly fixes everything. We have to be willing to try solutions that have worked for others and see if they are a good fit for our situation.

So while acknowledging that the emotional contributors to becoming overweight are many; let's look at it from the physical side. Once the obvious culprits are eliminated, you may want a more precise idea of how many calories you or your child needs. One of the biggest keys in a successful diet, be it for fat loss, muscle gain, recomposition, or even overall health is caloric balance. As we've already discussed, there are many factors related to changing or maintaining body composition but physically they all come down to simple energy balance.

A calorie is a unit of energy that is a representation of food energy utilized by the body. In order for successful weight loss to occur, there needs to be a deficit in caloric intake versus expenditure. There are several methods to give a rough idea of what an individual's caloric balance point will be. Use these as a starting point to see if you feel good on this amount of food and if you begin to lose weight.

Don't overlook feeling good especially when it comes to your child. I assure you, there are enough healthy food choices within your caloric needs that you do not need to suffer deprivation, weakness, light-headedness, and the rest. It's counterproductive to your goal of making a change that will last.

Metabolism is "the sum of the physical and chemical processes in an organism by which its material substance is produced, maintained, and destroyed, and by which energy is made available". There are three primary components involved in metabolism that provide measurable uses of energy. The first is Resting Metabolic Rate which is the energy requirement necessary for maintaining organ health, breathing, repairing the body, and thinking. RMR is responsible for approximately 60-70% of overall metabolic demand.

The second component of metabolism is responsible for another 20-25%. It's the amount of energy utilized by the body in performing activities. This can be your morning exercise routine or tennis match but it also includes routine activity, even brushing your teeth.

Finally, the remaining 10-15% comes from the energy required to digest and metabolize the food we eat. The Thermic Effect of Food varies. For example, it is easy for the body to digest fat and convert it into a usable substance. The body doesn't release much heat energy in this process. Protein, on the other hand, is harder for the body to convert to usable energy. There are several metabolic steps, each requiring some energy, which a protein must go through before it can provide energy. Some fibrous carbs, such as celery, may actually cost nearly as much energy to digest as they provide.

There are several methods that can give a good starting point for determining caloric need. I would strongly urge you to get the help of your pediatrician or a nutritionist to determine this for your growing child. I'd give the same advice to you but if you want a quick idea for an adult, you could use this formula as a starting point. Just remember to adjust according to results and to how you feel.

Men: Body Weight multiplied 12-15
Women: Body Weight multiplied 10-12

This is obviously not precise but acceptable because we are just looking for a starting place. Ingesting just 100 calories a day more than you need will result in about a ten pound weight gain over the course of a year. So this is nothing more than a ball park figure to use as a starting place. If you prefer to start with a custom designed starting point planned specifically for you, please consult your physician or a nutritionist.

Try this amount of food and make adjustments in 100-200 calorie increments until you find the amount that allows you to slowly and safely lose while feeling energetic and emotionally satisfied. Everyone's metabolism is different and a formula can't account for all the potential factors involved. Try adding menopause or hypothyroidism or a history of dieting to the mix. Be patient. Small permanent changes are much better than dramatic changes that overwhelm you into quitting.

So give the formula a try or alternatively, step away from the coke and tub of popcorn and see if you start to lose. We generally know what to do; it's doing it that's so hard. Still, if you suspect you are just over-consuming even healthy foods these numbers may be useful in determining how much you need to cut back.

Happily, the increased activity of the daily Exercising Values routine is going to burn some of those extra calories anyway. Just remember the maxim you cannot override a bad diet simply by training. It takes some attention to both calories in and calories out.

Different diets work for different people. Everyone needs protein, fats, carbohydrates, vitamins, minerals, and water but the precise ratios can vary. Research is showing that some of these variances can be quite dramatic. Once you determine your basic protein, fat, and fiber needs; you can add in carbs as activity level dictates, giving first consideration to the vitamins and minerals they contain.

For the less active, frequent feedings of large amounts of low-fiber carbs with nothing else will promote frequent blood sugar spikes. So including small amounts of protein rich foods with carbs is a good idea. The more active individual needs more carbs both for the energy they provide and for the water they store. They may find too few carbs will effect athletic performance.

Again, use general guidelines and adjust according to what you observe. My main concern when you're picking a plan to control calories is that you don't neglect nutrition. Proper food choices are the backbone of good health. Enjoyment is also important. It doesn't do a whole lot of good to follow a diet for a few months, lose weight, and then go right back to the way you were before because you disliked the food you were eating.

Certain foods should be avoided period. These include trans fats and high fructose corn syrup. HFCS increases appetite and offers no nutritional value. Trans fats have been linked to diabetes and clogged arteries that lead to heart disease and strokes. When trans fats enter your body they revert back to their solid state right inside your arteries. When reading labels, look for words such as hydrogenated, partially hydrogenated, or shortening, all code words for trans fat.

At least cut back on processed foods and foods with a high sugar content. If you need a little incentive consider this: sugary, starchy foods cause an inflammatory response that results in the glycation of collagen in the skin and all other organs. This lays the foundation for the beginning of wrinkles and sagging muscles. This loss of tone, elasticity and resilience effect your appearance. It is not the fine lines and wrinkles that give the face an aged appearance so much as it is the muscles in the face beginning to sag. Drooping muscles are the classic sign of an aging face and poor food choices spur it on.

Knowing that what we eat can help determine how young or old we look, we should replace that excessive sugar with a protein and antioxidant rich diet. Protein stimulates cells to repair themselves. Since we cannot store protein in our body, we must take in high quality protein every day to prevent the body from feeding upon itself by breaking down both tissue and muscle. When this happens, we lose the crisp jawline and our face takes on a soft doughy appearance especially when we are also consuming too much sugar.

Be selective as to what you put in your body. Like sugar, alcohol is also not your friend when it comes to weight loss. Preservatives and additives will neither preserve you nor add anything to your life. Be as vigilant as you can be for just a few weeks and these foods will lose their hold on you. If you have a known allergy by all means don't eat these inflaming foods even if they are healthy for someone without an allergy. Most people are drawn to the very foods they are allergic to but once you get them out of your system you'll find it easier to avoid them.

When your family associates better food choices with happy times with you; you give them an advantage that will last a lifetime. When your children are adults, these healthy foods are the ones they will turn to to calm down or feel better. Or perhaps they'll just go for a walk or do one of the workouts they remember doing with you as a child. Fun doesn't have to mean junk food even if everyone else is doing it. A cookie doesn't equal love unless you present it to your children as such.

Associations are very powerful determinants of behavior. Take charge and purposely create wholesome associations. This is more important than pushing so hard you end up injured or burned out. This program is for the long term so gradual progress will get you where you want to go. The journey in this case is every bit as important as the destination. So let's get ready to get started with the daily program.

CHAPTER TEN
FINAL GETTING STARTED TIPS

The Exercising Values program is divided into monthly segments. Each monthly program is built around four distinct character qualities and four fun family workouts. Let's take a look at this first month which you can use as a template to design your own program each month. Alternatively, for a nominal sum you can sign-up for online monthly updates to the program which will do all the planning for you. This will leave you with fresh workouts and updated fitness information on a regular basis.

Comprehensive Fitness

There are nine valuable components of fitness that Exercising Values addresses. We will naturally and significantly improve them in ourselves and in our children as we work through the daily exercises.

These essential pillars of physical fitness are:

Muscular Strength
This refers to the maximum strength a muscle or muscle group can generate at one time as the muscle exerts force against resistance. In Exercising Values, we use our body weight to build muscular strength.

Muscular Endurance
This is defined as the ability of a muscle or group of muscles to perform sustained work. By doing whole body exercises such as mountain climbers to fatigue, we work on muscular endurance.

Cardiovascular Endurance
This is the heart's ability to deliver blood to working muscles. By minimizing or eliminating the rest periods between exercises, we are able to work on cardiovascular endurance. Cardiovascular fitness will enhance all other forms of fitness as well as make daily activities easier and more enjoyable.

Strength Endurance

This is the muscle's ability to perform a maximum contraction continuously. An example would be repeated explosive jumping from the squat position.

Power

This is the ability to exert maximum muscular contraction instantaneously such as jumping as high or as far as you can.

Agility

An example of this is repeatedly making explosive movements in opposing directions such as bounding side to side in a zig zag pattern.

Balance

This involves controlling movement often on an unstable surface, such as if you were to stand on one foot.

Flexibility

This important ability requires achieving an extended range of motion and will help keep you looking younger and feeling better.

Coordination
When we put together the other eight elements it leads to a smooth execution of movement. An athlete is born.

Flexibility Training

Let's just look at flexibility as an example of how you will work on these nine elements during your Exercising Values session. Flexibility training is achieved through stretching. Make a habit of luxuriously stretching while still in bed in the morning and then when you first stand up. Bask in a few moments of self-care before you take on the world. Let this simple act remind you to take care of yourself all day long. Stretching is important for many reasons including:

To increase muscle length.
To enhance performance.

To reduce the pain associated with muscle and joint stiffness.

To move with a more youthful gait.

To improve posture.

To aid the healing of injured tissues and maintain previous range of motion.

To prevent injury.

Two exercises introduced in Exercising Values, "reaching for the moon" and "the lawn mower", are examples of dynamic stretching. An advantage to this type of stretching is that as it involves continuous movement it maintains warmth in the muscles. Additionally, it stimulates the nervous system and this particularly benefits children who are still developing coordination. Plus, it's fun to do.

The partner stretches and neck down total body stretching routine we will be doing are examples of static stretching. Static stretching involves applying sustained pressure to a muscle or muscle group in a lengthened position. A partner may allow you to find a deeper range of motion but these can be done alone.

Finally, there is PNF or "Proprioceptive Neuromuscular Facilitation". That mouthful just refers to combining a series of isometric contractions and static stretches. While very relaxing, they can take a bit of time to do, are harder to do on your own and are a bit more involved to learn properly. So it's a good idea to get some formal training before trying this on anyone. If you happen to have such training, it is fine to add it to the cool down but we will be focusing on the static and dynamic stretches that anyone, even beginners, can do.

Our concern is maintaining general flexibility so consistency is paramount. We want to make stretching a habit for everyone in the family. It can and should be done throughout the day but it should also have a time slot of its own.

Research on stretching is on-going and what was once considered common practice is increasingly being questioned. Holding static stretches longer that a few seconds has been found to reduce the gains of a workout designed to increase power. Static stretching right before going to the starting line is no longer recommended. Today, when I go to a competition, triathletes are warming up by running, biking, swimming, and doing related dynamic stretches but they are not doing static stretching until after the race, if at all.

Your goals as well as the time you have to devote to stretching influence what you do to get the most benefits. You can make your routine fit your schedule and still get results.

Muscles stretched for thirty seconds four to five times a day continue to increase their range of motion for six weeks before plateauing. If even that small amount of time is hard to find, relax. Muscles stretched for fifteen seconds four to five times a day can reach this same level. It will just take ten weeks instead of six.

Youth has its advantages. Your children won't have the stiffness that characterizes most adults. Encourage them to stretch now so it will become a habit like flossing or brushing their teeth. Make a game of it. Let them enjoy the fact that they are probably more flexible than you are. Acknowledge this with praise now and you may motivate them to keep that flexibility their entire lives.

I need you to understand that research may prove some of these suggestions wrong over time. There are always new discoveries where optimal performance is concerned. I do not intend to bog you down with the research but I want to assure you that my recommended workouts will always reflect current knowledge.

For this reason, I have created a monthly membership program for families that are interested in receiving additional workouts that incorporate the latest research findings. These updates also include additional character lessons, parenting tips and mom's moments. This resource serves to encourage mothers to meet their own goals as well as their family's goals.

For now, the available research supports using static stretches to achieve short-term range-of-motion gains. By holding these stretches for fifteen to thirty seconds and by repeating each stretch 4 or 5 times you will achieve increased flexibility that will last one to two hours. For long-term improvement choose the higher end thirty seconds and continue to do each stretch four or five times. You'll see improvement in about six weeks. Dynamic stretching is preferable before activity but static stretching can be an important part of the cool down since warm muscles respond better to the demands placed on them.

Ten Exercise Tips

In sports training there is the concept of the breakthrough workout. This means that a workout is designed to go a bit beyond what you usually demand of yourself. By definition, these involve more time to recover, usually at least 36 hours. Although some recent research found that women may recover much quicker from workouts than men.

One study found that women were recovering in four hours whereas it took men a full forty-eight hours. Pay attention to how long it takes you to recover and rest when needed. Workouts tear down and it is actually during recovery that we grow stronger. The more intensely you work, the more recovery time you may need.

Friday is the perfect time in the week to do a breakthrough workout. Elite athletes center their training around their breakthrough workouts and it is a good concept to introduce to the young aspiring athlete. It will also boost your own fitness. It prevents acclimating to your workouts which can reduce your calorie burn. It keeps everything more challenging and more fun.

If your typical day includes sleeping, eating, driving, watching T.V., working at a computer or studying behind a desk then you may be spending at least twenty of your twenty-four hours lying down or sitting. So simply, this tip is to stand up. Brief breaks from sitting will leave you feeling more refreshed and, believe it or not, will over time improve your overall fitness.

There is a reason we all have a negative association with the term coach potato. Stay glued to the coach and you'll soon be able to do little else. Studies show that an obese person is more likely to ask someone else to fetch them a drink whereas a fit person will naturally get up and get it themselves. Unless you are recovering from major surgery, are nursing a baby, have a broken leg or the flu; try to be self-sufficient and look for excuses to move.

Pay attention to early signs of getting sick. Don't suppress your immune system by training too hard on a day you need it to fight an infection. Once you have a fever you can expect the virus to be everywhere including in your muscles. So rest. Just because we have a harder than usual workout planned doesn't mean you have to do it. Save it for a day you are feeling 100%.

Frequent infections definitely need to be addressed in case a food allergy or lifestyle choice is making it worse. As a child, I took in a lot of second-hand smoke before the dangers of that were known and consequently I had chronic allergies. There are likely other dangers that are not yet fully understood. For example, plastic bottles are increasingly being linked to various health problems.

Stress can also be a factor so think about anything unusual that is happening at school or at home. Reduce your stress and you may reduce your sick days.

Commit to your program. It's important not to abandon the daily Exercising Values routine when you encounter a time of busyness or stress. One ten year study compared a group that consistently exercised mildly but very consistently to a group that exercised intensely but sporadically. They found that the first group had 68% better results than the less consistent group in spite of their more demanding routine.

Encourage each other. Working out with other people yields about 43% faster results and who better to work out with than those with whom you live. Successful people always surround themselves with other positive, successful people. The first character quality we talk about in the Exercising Values program is enthusiasm for that very reason.

Hang out with positive people who take action and don't whine or complain about it. That alone will go a long way to assuring you of success. Teach your child to be the kind of person who attracts other successful, responsible people and peer pressure will never be an issue.

Keep the family interested. Our exercise time will be loosely structured. Children's attention spans vary greatly. Rather than trying to impose specific time limits for each exercise just relax and move from one to the next as seems natural. Think play time rather than workout. Within this flexible outlook we'll aim to keep this special time to about fifteen to twenty minutes.

If you have a limitation or injury work around it rather than aggravating it. For example, if you can't do mountain climbers just continue vigorously doing the movements from the warm-up. You can always substitute a movement from the warm-up for an exercise you need to skip. Do keep moving. You should consult your doctor if you have any questions about the suitability of an exercise for you.

Include rest. Include laughter. Try not to approach this time as something on a to do list to be marked off. Once your children know that they have your undivided attention for a special portion of the day, they may take advantage of it by sharing with you what's on their hearts and minds.

Consistency Trumps Duration

Be content with short consistent daily sessions. Believe me, this is critical to your success. You are making a change. Consistency is your best friend when trying to establish a habit. When life throws you surprises: illness, a major project at work or school, house guests,or whatever; an hour commitment would seem daunting and frankly is unlikely to happen. But fifteen or twenty minutes seems doable. Really, who can't find fifteen minutes in their day to:

- Build strong family relationships
- Improve health and fitness
- Make weight management easier

- Instill values in their children
- Open the lines of communication between generations and among siblings
- De-stress
- Laugh
- Have fun!

Short Workouts Get Big Results

While you are investing in your children you will also be doing some wonderful things for your own body. At times, these short workouts can be very intense. Research has shown that when working at a higher heart rate, you will burn more calories both during the workout and for up to 24 hours afterward. This after-burn helps you toward the goal of more fat-burning lean body mass.

Your skin will also benefit from exercise. Sweat eliminates many toxins from the body. It also improves circulation to the skin which gives you an attractive, healthy glow while decreasing the development of wrinkles. When the skin of athletes is examined under a microscope their skin is thicker with more and healthier collagen to give the skin strength, flexibility, and a more youthful appearance. Just because you are a mom doesn't mean you need to look as tired as you sometimes feel.

If you always do the same exercises your body will adapt to them and over time you will not get as much calorie burning from your sessions. This will never happen with the Exercising Values program because I have manipulated the exercise variables for you from week to week. In addition, we are using some of the latest research to get maximum results in minimum time.

For example, while doing total body exercises, we alternate the emphasis between upper and lower body because this forces our heart to pump the blood to the working muscles in what is known as peripheral heart action. Research shows, by alternating in this fashion, you will actually burn up to twice as many calories. It will also help you keep up your intensity which will lead to better muscle development. Because you are switching muscle groups, very little rest will be needed between exercises. This will elevate your heart, add excitement for the kids, and will help you continue to burn fat even when the short workout is over.

Some studies have shown that by performing your abdominal work when the body is already warm you may actually burn more belly fat. This contradicts the long held belief that spot reduction is impossible. Research in exercise science is constant. This controversy will be resolved, challenged, and then re-challenged. You'll want to stay on top of research like that. The online Exercising Values program will keep you on the cutting edge of what is most effective because it is updated month by month with research, new workouts, more character qualities, and more support for moms.

There are some simple assessments you can do if you'd like to monitor your progress. Children may enjoy these but they should never be used to make a child feel like he is not measuring up to an unreachable standard. Some of the intangible improvements can't really be measured but you'll notice improvements in energy, happiness, and yes, in enthusiasm for the fit lifestyle.

How Hard To Work

The effectiveness of short workouts comes from their intensity but it is ill-advised to jump into high intensity right away. Even if your cardiovascular system and muscles can handle the stress, you must be sure that connective tissue and your nervous system as a whole has a chance to adapt. So don't push too hard in the beginning weeks.

On a scale from one to ten, your perceived exertion should be around a five or six if you are new to exercise and around a six or seven if you have already been active for at least six to eight weeks. Over time, you will build to an eight which represents a high end, predominantly aerobic workout rather than a lung and leg burning predominantly anaerobic nine or ten. In other words, while it will be challenging, it will be doable and not unpleasant. If for some reason you are planning a longer workout, then these levels should be lower.

A more precise way to look at it would be to consider the research on maximum fat burning. In a series of recent studies, the exercise intensity at which maximal fat burning was observed was 50% of VO2 max in a group of untrained individuals and was 62-63% of VO2 max or 70-75% of heart rate max for trained individuals. These are low and moderate intensity levels respectively. Other factors affecting fat burning include the duration of the exercise, the mode of exercise, gender differences, nutritional supplements, diet and environmental factors such as temperature.

A good rule of thumb is to stay at a level that will allow you to come back tomorrow. Consistent action is going to do more for you than one heroic effort that takes days from which to recover. Once you have adapted to the program, you'll have a chance to increase your normal level of exertion on breakthrough Friday. We may even go for a perceived exertion of nine or ten during the breakthrough workout.

Working out should have an ebb and flow to it rather than driving 100% all the time. Progress actually occurs while you are resting and rebuilding not during the actual workout. Train smart. Listen to your body. When in doubt, back off or do less. Your intensity will naturally rise over time and by then you'll have made exercise a habit.

The Workout Area

You need to find a place within your house or yard where everyone can move about without breaking or running into anything. So clear a little space ahead of time. Home school families may be more inclined than most to think of the alphabet as a decorative tool or the multiplication tables as something to be hung on the door. My home for many years had a balance beam, a set of parallel bars in the library, a Fisher Price basketball hoop and an easel in the family room. Books were everywhere. Let's just say that a visitor could tell that children lived there.

That arrangement wouldn't suit everyone and I'm not particularly advocating it for you. But I will say it sent a message to my children that there is more to do come evening time than plop in front of the television. Happily, Exercising Values requires no equipment or dedication of space so stay within your own comfort zone. By all means, when the weather is nice feel free to take this outdoors. If you have the space, occasionally changing rooms might add interest. Basements, garages and apartment common areas might provide possibilities.

A Great Beginning

This is it. Unless you still need to discuss your exercise or diet plan with your doctor, you have everything you need to begin. Please don't delay. Getting started is the hardest part but once you do you are setting yourself and your children up for success. As a personal trainer, I've seen many sedentary people become devoted exercisers mostly because it made them feel terrific and also because of the results they saw.

I'm excited for you. Post comments on my blog www.exercisingvalues.com/blog or e-mail me at pamdavenport@exercisingvalues.com I'd love to hear about your successes and to help you through any obstacles. Thank you for being a part of Exercising Values.

CHAPTER ELEVEN
THE EXERCISING VALUES DAILY PROGRAM

Week One - Day One

Just like we are easing into our new program we want to ease into and out of each workout. It is important not to skip the warm-up and cool down. It would be better to do fewer sets of the main workout. We want to avoid injury and prepare the body for intensity. It's important to teach these aspects of athletic training. Your children will see them again if they become involved in organized sports. All serious athletes warm-up and cool down and so should you. Besides they are fun to do.

Warm-Up for Week One - Day One

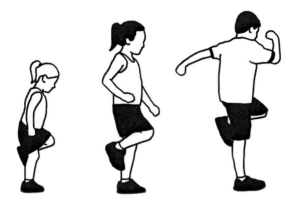

Begin with a march but keep your feet close to the floor and your arms by your side. Next advance to a regular march and move your arms as well. Finally, do an exaggerated march with your arms swinging high into the air. Now do all three sizes again but this time add a little bounce to your movements.

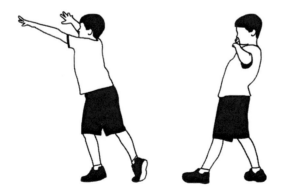

Now we're going to reach for the moon so put one foot in front of the other and rock back and forth as if you were a rocking horse. As you rock forward, reach for the sky with both hands and then pull back your prize by bringing both elbows in and back. Do this several times. Change which foot is in front and repeat.

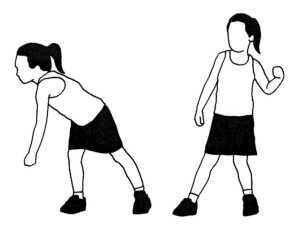

One job kids can help with is yard work so to get ready to help out we'll mimic the starting of a lawn mower. Stand with your feet apart in a straddle. Now bend and reach to one side by the floor and past your foot. Pull back and up like you were starting a lawn mower. Repeat a few times and then change sides and do it all again.

Introducing the Character Quality

Warmed up and ready to work it's time to announce the character quality of the day:

ENTHUSIASM

Enthusiasm is intense and eager enjoyment, interest, or approval.

We want to keep it simple so we launch right into the workout after announcing the character quality and one of its definitions. In the sections following the warm-up each day, you'll find additional information and ideas for you to teach to your children and to ponder yourself as you strive to model and teach enthusiasm. Work these ideas into conversation either during the workout, the story time, around the dinner table, or any other teachable moment.

If you put these ideas in your heart and mind they will find a way into your words and into your life. So there is no need to read it aloud or go over it formally with your kids. Soon enough everyone in the family will be expanding their concept of enthusiasm as it naturally unfolds during your time together.

To Share with the Family

Everyone appreciates the enthusiastic person who is eager to spread their good cheer. They approach each task with a willingness to work hard without complaining. Their upbeat attitude is contagious and they make hard jobs fun for others. Enthusiasm enables us to bring our best to a task.

At the beginning of any improvement we are attempting to make, there will be a natural enthusiasm. It is also natural for this enthusiasm to wane when we are presented with the inevitable obstacles. Character involves choosing to remain enthusiastic when complaining or getting discouraged seems like the easier choice. Good character always involves choice.

Parent's Points to Ponder

You may have wondered why with all the character qualities to choose from I chose to begin our program with enthusiasm. Approaching a task or a lifestyle change with enthusiasm is a step toward guaranteeing successful completion of that task or change. Even more important is the effect enthusiasm has on others. Since this is a family project, it seemed right to start with a quality that naturally spreads it's good effects to others in the family.

Enthusiasm helps ensure that everyone will give their best effort and that is what we are seeking. Remember Exercising Values is an invitation to a party not something we want anyone to do begrudgingly or half-heartedly. So offer lots of praise to show that you notice and appreciate when your children are trying hard with an upbeat attitude.

Workout for Week One - Day One

Now that we are warmed up and have today's character quality in mind; it's time to start the workout. It takes a lot of determination and enthusiasm to make it up a mountain. Our first exercise is called mountain climbers.

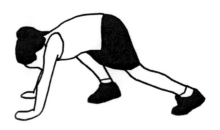

Begin with your hands and feet on the floor like you are about to do a push-up. Now bend one knee and bring that foot forward. With a jumping motion we'll change which leg is bent in front and which one is straightened out behind. Keep switching legs up to one minute or until you are tired. Then return to your starting position.

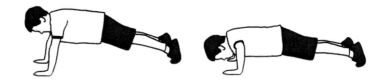

Next are push-ups and if you can do them from your hands and feet that's great. Another choice would be to drop to your knees.

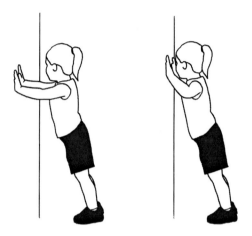

If you prefer you can stand up and lean into a wall and do your push-ups that way. Someday you may want to place your feet up on a chair to make your push-up harder. Go down slowly while you count to four then explode up like a kernel of popcorn popping. It is better for your shoulders if you stop when you are about the size of your fist from the floor rather than going all the way down. In about one minute or when you get tired, you are ready to move on.

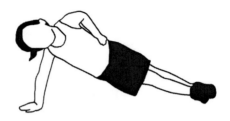

Now we want you on your side with your legs extended and your feet stacked one on top of the other. You can choose to support yourself on your forearm or you can rise up onto your hand with your arm straight but not locked out. Keep the other hand on your hip. Hold this side plank about thirty seconds or until you get tired and then switch sides and repeat. Now you just have one more exercise to go!

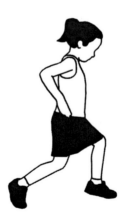

Remember the marching we did during our warm-up? Now we are going to take a giant step forward and you'll want to lift your leg high just like you did in the exaggerated march. Then step as far forward as you can, bending your knee as you finish. Lower your body slowly and then spring back to your standing position. Change legs and do it again. One time on each leg may do it but you can keep switching legs until you are tired. We call this exercise the lunge.

If time permits and you and your family want to, you may repeat this series one, two or even three more times.

Cool Down for Week One - Day One

For the cool down, we will repeat the first part of the warm-up without the bouncing movements. So once again march but keep your feet close to the floor and your arms by your side. Next, advance to a regular march and move your arms as well. Finally do an exaggerated march with your arms swinging high into the air. We'll skip the intensity raising bounces this time and move right to reaching for the moon and lawn mower stretches which you'll want to do two or three times each.

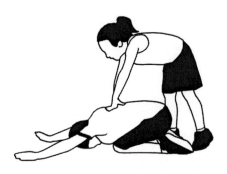

Now we'll end with a partner stretch which is a great way to show kindness to each other and reward each other for a job well done. A simple one is for one person to kneel down with their bottom on their heels and reach as far forward as they can while looking straight down at the floor. When they can't reach any further forward their partner will slowly and gently push first on the middle of their back and then on the top of their back to help their partner reach just a bit further.

Small children may even sit on their parent's back instead of pushing. Either way, this assisted stretch will feel great and you can switch places and return the favor. You'll feel tired but relaxed as we conclude.

Character Classics: A Follow-up Activity for Character Building

Exercising Values is more than a program of family fun through exercise and character lessons. I also recommend sharing with your children well-loved, timeless stories that illustrate the featured character quality. If you have time after your workout, you could begin an appropriate story from children's literature that will illustrate enthusiasm. Otherwise, save it as a separate activity for later in the day. Some families may have time to do it all in the morning and others might want to save the story as part of a bedtime routine.

Too much of what is presented to children is dumbed down. Take a look at what the American founding fathers and others of that era were reading at an early age and how advanced it is, what you find may very well astound you. So don't be too concerned that a wisely chosen book will be too difficult for your children. They can understand books that are read to them long before they might be able to read the book on their own. Condensed versions are an option but I am confident your child will have no trouble with the excerpts.

It is fun to discover how character traits are illustrated in great literature. The beloved novel, Pollyanna, by Eleanor H. Porter touches everyone because of the cheerful enthusiasm of the title character. In Pollyanna, we find the famous phrase: 'if we look for the bad, expecting it; we will find it." Pollyanna, on the other hand, chooses to be enthusiastic and to look for the good in life. Modern films are still made based on this engaging character created in 1913.

Another classic story that shows the effect enthusiasm has on others is Mark Twain's book Tom Sawyer. You may recall the story where Tom gets his friends to help him white wash a fence by showing enthusiasm for the task rather than complaining. It is mainly the story of Tom's persuading his friends that speaks to the power of enthusiasm.

Tom Sawyer is better suited to older children. This story can lead to a valuable discussion about peer pressure, how to treat friends, and the ethical use of our own powers of persuasion. Younger children might just enjoy hearing what Tom's friends are pulling out of their pockets to barter with Tom.

Recordings of the excerpts as well as complete versions of each novel are also available at www.exercisingvalues.com. The full novels are intended for families with children who are ready for them but the excerpt alone will do a good job of causing your children to reflect on the featured character quality.

The website is there to support you while you move forward with your Exercising Values program. The blog is a resource for parenting and exercise tips. Feel free to post questions and share your experiences. The monthly Exercising Values program is available and parallels the daily program in this book. In addition to all new workouts and character lessons, the monthly program also includes recordings of excerpts from each month's character classic, mom's moments, and parenting tips.

Character Challenge

After the workout or story you will want to leave your family with a challenge to apply what they've learned. For example, you can ask them to determine to show enthusiasm while performing a routine task today. Suggest that they set out to make the other people involved in the task more motivated and happier by their example.

Enthusiasm is contagious so the family can see how many people they can spread it to today. When you tell your family how you inspired others, that will motivate them, too. Tom got the whole neighborhood to help him with a tiresome task just by showing enthusiasm. Now let's see what you can do.

As you might expect, teaching and reinforcing good character with our children has been shown to improve our own character. We are making a serious commitment to be good role models. We will want to make a special effort to demonstrate the character trait and to talk to our children about our efforts. Don't be afraid to talk about your failures as much as your successes.

For example, it was my son and not me that displayed a servant's heart in this story. I had been called for jury duty. The case involved a young man of 22 who was being tried for a crime he may have committed several years ago. Straight out of college, I used to work with juvenile felons. I tried to help them find their way to a different life. Believe me, I have stories. It's probably because of my previous work with juvenile offenders that I was passed over for serving that day.

I'll admit I was relieved. While I was listening to the attorneys sort through our qualifications to serve, there was some place I would rather have been. My oldest son, Dane, was on his way to the airport to pick up my middle son, Skyler. Skyler had spent about a month doing some volunteer work in Taiwan. I was anxious to see him and hear about his adventures. He had been with a team working in the Character

Institute with children whose parents were attending the Basic Seminar, an outreach of the Institute in Basic Life Principles.

At the time, all three of my sons were vegetarians; all three of my daughters were not. The boys started when they were quite young. So we were all amazed to learn that while there Skyler temporarily gave up being a vegetarian. He bit the head off shrimp, ate squid and a number of other things the meat eaters in the family wouldn't touch. Upon returning home, he went right back to his vegetarian ways but he said he wanted the full cultural experience while he was there. Dane noted the irony that it was the non-vegetarians who were most shocked by what Skyler choked down and mostly enjoyed.

It was wonderful to hear about the children he had worked with and the friendships he had made. Skyler has a soft heart for children. The night Skyler returned from Taiwan that soft heart benefited me. We were all sitting around the family room together because my oldest daughter, Jennifer, and her eighteen month old son, Daniel, were visiting us.

Daniel hadn't been feeling well and when my grandson threw up it was Skyler, still suffering from jet lag, that sprang into action; cleaning up his nephew and the couch. He looked at it and was as disgusted as anyone would be but he took care of it anyway.

That's Skyler in a nutshell. He'll do what needs to be done, nonchalantly and good-naturedly. It's moments like those when you see your children not only go off to try to make a difference in the world but who are also willing to do the unpleasant but necessary daily jobs; that you realize that children are a blessing from the Lord. These days I learn a lot from the children I spent years teaching.

Although we parents want to be good role models please don't think to convey these truths to your children that you have to be stellar examples of each character quality. I was sitting on the other side of my grandson when he threw up and I was thinking: throw up? I don't see any throw up. Not much enthusiasm, loyalty, diligence or hospitality on display from my reaction. This was not my finest moment.

Sometimes it is more powerful to admit to being a bad example. If you are trying to teach about enthusiasm and the whole family saw you grumbling about picking up after them or cleaning the garage or whatever, then just say so. Tell them that you are purposing to do better next time and then try to follow-through. It gives them permission to not be perfect. Believe it or not, when they see you making an effort but struggling to be enthusiastic about doing an unpleasant job; they will remember the character lesson you were trying to teach.

I've always thought one of the values of spending time with your children is they get to see you wrestle with things. They get to see you fail. They get to see you try again. Your faith and your values are not something they hear about but rather something they see you trying to apply; undoubtedly with mixed results.

It's great to have lots of time to get this done but not everyone has that luxury. I've had seasons in my life where my time with my children was also limited. That's when it becomes even more important to make the most of the time we do have.

I really believe these short daily fifteen minute lessons that are attached to fun physical activity will lay a solid foundation for children that they will remember and apply. Exercising Values can easily be expanded upon to provide a physical education program for home-educated students. I hope that many home-schooling families will find it useful. But I also wanted to get it in the hands of parents who are working or have other obligations that limit their time with their family. I hope it is helpful to families who want to maximize the time they do have together.

The attorneys were wise in not choosing me to serve on the jury that day. Even though I thought I could be impartial and render a verdict just on the evidence; I did have a heart for the young man on trial that day. I wondered how he got there. I wondered who had tried or not tried to teach him right from wrong.

Not every character flaw will land us in jail but all character flaws make us less effective, they grieve our Maker, they hurt other people. The character challenge gives parents as well as children a chance to reflect on whether or not they demonstrate that character quality in their lives and to take action to improve.

Mom's Moment

After each workout I like to take just a minute to speak to moms. Ever heard, "when momma ain't happy ain't nobody happy." It's not great English, but nonetheless it holds a great truth. So my encouragement to you is to take just five minutes today to sit in a relaxing chair, take a few deep breaths and take just a moment to visualize the changes you'd like to see in your family. The ones that, in fact, will make you happy. Picture it as clearly and with as much detail as you can. Close your eyes if it helps you concentrate.

Discover what you value most for your children. I want to help you reach that vision. I'll be your personal trainer and I'll take the guesswork out of creating a time-efficient exercise routine suitable for the whole family. I'll add structure to your hopes and dreams to teach and model good character. Like a good neighbor or friend, I'd like the opportunity to lend support to your good intentions and help you be successful.

If you are beginning to capture a vision of how your family will benefit from daily time together doing a short exercise session and talking about good character then keep that picture in your mind on a daily basis. Remember the expected benefits. Realize that to get them you need to take consistent action. Besides five minutes of relaxed focus will be good for you.

Set aside just a few moments to enjoy that you have taken action to improve your family's health and well-being. Exercising Values will have an impact in preventing obesity, diabetes, heart disease, and osteoporosis. It will have a hand in bringing out your child's athletic potential. This foundation will lead to a lifetime of better health and fitness.

In Proverbs 4 there is a promise that doing the right thing will bring health to a man's whole body. As much as physical training does for our well-being; character training will do more. I hope that as you try the program with your family you will experience it's many benefits.

Week One - Day Two

On day one, we introduced the warm-up/cool down and four key exercises for week one. We also introduced the character quality of enthusiasm. For the remainder of the week we will build on that foundation offering slight variations to each exercise. Do not feel locked into adding variations if your family is still enjoying and mastering the initial workout. The pattern I am offering you is merely a suggestion of one way to organize your workout week but it can be adapted to your individual family's schedule.

Warm-Up for Week One - Day Two

We will follow the pattern we established on day one by beginning with small movements and progressing to exaggerated ones. On day one we began with a march and of course you could repeat that. But for variety, I suggest you change the movement to a front kick. Begin small, build to a higher kick and finish with the highest kick you can do. You'll need to spread out a bit so no one gets hurt.

Next, let's go through the three sizes of kicks again adding ballistic movements. So now you are jumping from one foot to the next with a kick. Reach for the moon a few times and then finish with a few lawn mowers and we should be warm and ready to go.

To Share with the Family

Immediately following the warm-up, we briefly repeat that enthusiasm is the character quality of the week. Challenge everyone to do the workout with enthusiasm. We'll transition into the main workout from the warm-up by doing a quick drill to work on balance and proprioception. Each person will be asked to identify simple words associated with enthusiasm. If you have trouble coming up with a list consider:

1. Smile
2. Energy
3. Fun
4. Happy

Each person will use their body to spell out the word while others guess what it is. Trace the letters with your foot or form the letters with your arms or body. Be creative. This can be done standing on one foot or for the ultimate challenge on one foot with both eyes closed. Older children could also spell enthusiasm.

This balance training will strengthen your core and children will probably enjoy the fact that they usually have much better balance than their parents. Be ready to be a good sport if they laugh at you as you hop around attempting to keep your equilibrium.

Research in exercise psychology show that adults and children have more fun when mere fitness activities are made into a challenge or a game. These studies also show that feeling competent is the single best predictor of that enjoyment. Occasionally surpassing a parent is great fun for a child.

Parent's Points to Ponder

Striving for excellence is one thing, demanding it from beginners is another. Never overlook someone's efforts to do their best regardless of where they are in their skill development. Research shows that when children are only praised for achievement that they will tend to avoid difficult tasks and challenges and look for easy ways to get approval. On the other hand, when they are praised for character and effort they will seek out challenges and willingly work at difficult assignments.

Not every exercise will come easily and at times good form may take a while to learn. There is no failure, just steps toward improvement and eventual mastery. The process, while challenging, should be fun and uplifting. As a parent, you will see potential in your children long before they are able to recognize it in themselves. Let them know that you believe in them and see them as being successful.

Workout for Week One - Day Two

We'll begin with the familiar mountain climbers. Try to do a few more than yesterday. Happily, you will work the cardiopulmonary system, the chest, shoulders, lower abs and transversus abdominus. Remember we'll be repeating this exercise throughout the week and it will get easier.

Next we continue to work the chest, shoulders and abs while also targeting the triceps by returning to push-ups. This time go down on a count of two and back up on a count of two. Remember to stop when you are within the size of your fist rather than going all the way to the ground. This will protect your shoulders.

Now we move on to work the inner and outer obliques with side planks. This time we will try to add lifting the top leg into the air. Hold this for about thirty seconds or until you are tired and then switch sides.

Our last exercise is the lunge. This time we will lunge forward with one leg. As your foot hits the ground bend both knees until the forward leg is parallel to the floor and the back leg is perpendicular to it with the heel of the foot on that leg elevated off the floor. Push-up from the front foot and repeat until fatigued and then switch sides.

This works the glutes, hamstrings, and quads while working your cardiovascular system as well. If you like, you can repeat all four exercises again one or two more times before cool down.

Cool Down for Week One - Day Two

For cool down, we simply repeat the non-ballistic portions of the front kicks from the warm-up, do reach for the moon a few times and finish with a few lawn mowers. For our partner stretch, you will chose a partner about your same height or someone tall can kneel down facing a shorter partner. With arms straight, you will place your hand at the top of the inside of each others arm. Now turn and look away until you feel a good stretch in the chest. Now do the same thing with the other arm.

If time permits also do the partner stretch for your back from day one. Don't forget to give each other a big smile for another job well done.

Character Classics

If you haven't done so yet and time permits, you could listen to the character rich story, Pollyanna. Or you may prefer the story of how one boy, Tom Sawyer, got a hard job done by enticing others to help him through enthusiasm. If it fits your schedule better, save story reading for bedtime. Stories are a great way to reinforce ideas.

Character Challenge

Try to encourage people with a smile today. You may be surprised how differently people will react to you when you offer them this simple gesture of acceptance and caring. Remember the story of the man who tipped his hat for Desmond Tutu's mother and changed the course of history. Make someone's day by lighting up when you see them. Who knows but you, too, may set in motion a butterfly effect that one day impacts the world for good.

I have a friend who's a bit of a live wire. One day when we were driving to lunch with my daughter, he suddenly pulls the car over and runs into the store to fetch something one of us had said we needed. My daughter is giggling because he takes such sudden and abrupt action and in the process is being amazingly generous and kind. It wasn't his problem but he solved it anyway. But what I really remember about that day is what happened next.

We were stopped at a stoplight when looking down the hill up ahead he spots someone he knows who is stopped at a light on the cross street. So he gets out of the car and races down the hill, pounds on her window, waves and says hi and then dashes back up the hill before the light has changed. Okay, there may be some A.D.H.D. involved here but there is also a soul that makes other people, especially his young children, know they are seen and heard.

Think for a moment about anyone you know who exudes enthusiasm and I bet it makes you smile. I know this friend always does that for me. Your own young children can do that for you. I can always count on my enthusiastic little grandson, Daniel, to make me laugh. Make it your goal to brighten someone's day with your positive attitude.

Mom's Moment

Take those relaxing few moments to once again reflect on the results you are hoping to get from this program but this time I want you to think about yourself rather than just the children. Perhaps you want to lose some weight, feel more energetic or be more upbeat around your children. Try to picture exactly what the results you are looking for would look like. Imagine it in great detail.

Remember everyone in the family benefits when you take care of yourself. So take care of yourself inside and out. Be pretty. Have adventures. Most of all, be yourself.

Week One - Day Three

Warm-Up for Week One - Day Three

By now the pattern of our warm-up is familiar. We slightly vary the muscles used to keep it fresh and interesting. So today our front kicks become side kicks. We still start with small movements building first to average and then exaggerated movements. Then we will add the hop from side to side as we once again build from small movements to large. Finish with first a lawnmower or two on each side and then by reaching for the moon. Simply changing the order of exercises helps us progress.

To Share with the Family

Before we start the main exercises, we once again introduce enthusiasm. We will give each person a chance to share what they have noticed in their interactions with other people since making an effort to smile and to be more enthusiastic. Practice listening carefully to what each person says and try to say something encouraging about their efforts.

Parent's Points to Ponder

The world likes to label people. Be sure that the labels you give at home are success oriented like "you are such a great person to be around, I love your enthusiastic attitude!." Visualize success for them and express it. Base this on what you really do see. Sincerity is essential. Encourage them as much as you can.

Remember you are their coach and you want to inspire them to want to deliver their best. You are setting them up to be a good influence on others because people who get praise tend to give it. People who notice the good in others will always have a following.

Workout for Week One - Day Three

Encourage everyone to do their mountain climbers with gusto as we try to improve on what we did the day before.

Today we do our pushups to a 1/4 count. So we lower quickly and then take our time coming back up. This will require additional muscular strength.

Plank time. We are still working on the side plank but today we will try to lift the hand that was on our hip high into the air. This will require additional balance and core strength. Return to an easier level if you need to. Always keep it fun, not frustrating.

Yesterday we talked about moving more and that's just what we are going to do with our lunges. We will make them walking lunges. So alternate legs as you travel across the room and back or in a circle.

Cool Down for Week One - Day Three

Cool down with your side kicks, lawnmowers and by reaching for the moon. During cool down you may omit the side kicks with the hops to assist your heart rate in returning to normal. Now that we are settling in to a solid routine, it is time to expand on the post work out stretching. We began our first two sessions with a couple of fun partner stretches. Now we want to add a more comprehensive stretching routine to include all of the muscles we have been targeting. First let's cover a few of the basics.

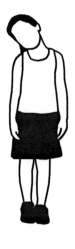

The Stretching Routine

We'll start with the neck and work our way down. Stand straight with your arms at your sides. Reach towards the floor with your finger tips and then move your head to one side for a count of thirty and then to the other side.

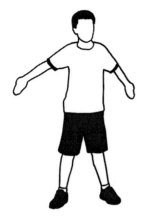 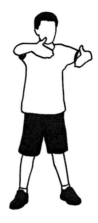

Now switch to a dynamic stretch by bringing your arms out to the side and then alternate between rounding the arms and back as though you were hugging a big tree and drawing your arms back and pushing the chest out. By alternating static stretches and dynamic stretches we can optimize our workout time.

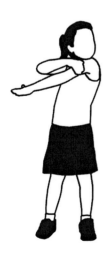

Now take one arm across the body and assist the stretch with your other arm just above or below the elbow of the stretching arm. After holding this for twenty to thirty seconds look over the shoulder of the arm you are not stretching while still holding on to your arm. Now return to the front and drop your shoulder down as you still hold onto your arm. This pattern will stretch first the shoulder, then the back and then will stretch the shoulder again in a slightly different way. This should be repeated on the other side.

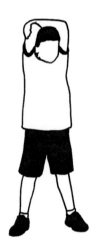

To stretch the triceps, bend your arm over your head and reach down your back. By placing the hand of your other arm just above the elbow of the stretching arm you may achieve a better stretch. Repeat on the other side, of course.

A wall or training partner can assist you with stretching your lower body. Placing one foot in front of the other, much like the beginning of a lunge, will allow you to lower the back heel towards the ground to stretch the calf. Then, if you shift your weight towards your back leg, you can lift the toes up and back on the front leg. By leaning over that leg you'll achieve a stretch for the hamstrings or back of the leg.

Holding on to the wall, a piece of furniture or your partner will allow you to then stretch the quads or front of the leg. This is done by bending your leg behind you, holding onto your ankle and gently pulling. When you release the leg cross it behind the other leg and lean to each side for an IT band stretch. Repeat with the other leg.

This is but a small sampling of possible stretches that within our time frame will give you good results. If you have the time to repeat them four or five times throughout the day, you will maximize those results.

Character Classics

Don't forget to spend some time seeing what Tom or Pollyanna are up to today even if it's just for a minute or two before bed.

Character Challenge

Move and stretch as often as you can throughout your day. Just do this in a spontaneous way, much as you naturally would do upon awakening. As you reach and stretch, let it remind you to do everything you do today with enthusiasm. In fact, see if you can influence someone else to move more or to stretch a bit. Your enthusiasm for your new habit will make others want to try it.

Mom's Moment

Take a pencil and paper and make a list of 5-10 goals you identified for your family or for yourself the past two days. Keep the list with you and read it a couple times during the day. At the end of the day, take just a few minutes to close your eyes and once again visualize how life will be better for you and your family when those dreams are a reality. Take pleasure in knowing you made progress towards that goal today.

Week One - Day Four

Warm-Up for Week One - Day Four

Now that everyone has had the opportunity to practice the push-up for a few days, let's use it to assess upper body strength. It will be fun to later repeat the test and see our improvement. Growing children have that added advantage and will see substantial change over time.

First, we want to go through our warm-up with today's kicks being straight legs to the back. Small to large and no impact to ballistic. Then a few dynamic stretches such as reaching for the moon and the lawn mower. While standing, mimic the motion of a push-up by reaching forward and then drawing the elbows back. Do this several times to begin to warm-up the chest and shoulders. Now we'll move on to an assessment of our upper body strength.

Partner up. From either the knees or the toes perform as many push-ups as you can without pausing or stopping. Your partner will help you count and record them with today's date. If you performed them from your toes, you were pressing approximately 75% of your weight and if you chose to do them from your knees, then you lifted about 60% of your body weight. If this proves to be too much, remember they can be done in an upright position against a wall.

Earlier we placed the average consecutive push-ups for children at 5-25 depending on age and gender. The standards for adults also vary by age. Excellent is more than 54 for someone in their twenties, more than 44 if in their thirties, more than 39 in their forties, more than 34 in their fifties and more than 29 in their sixties. However, the more important measure for children and adults is improvement over time to achieve a personal best.

To Share with the Family

Just a quick review of the character quality and its definition will do. Enthusiasm is intense and eager enjoyment, interest, or approval.

Parent's Points to Ponder

Your enthusiasm for your child's athletic potential will carry them through whenever they find an exercise complicated or strenuous. Be patient yourself and show approval when an older sibling helps a younger one. Foster an atmosphere of teamwork and family unity.

Don't just praise performance, praise character and concern for others. You don't need to lower the standard of what mastery looks like but recognize the steps toward its achievement. Be a discouragement buster! Help them understand that every sprinter once took baby steps and they will make progress, too. For the same reasons, avoid being self-critical as well.

Workout for Week One - Day Four

Immediately following the push-up test, begin mountain climbers. They may seem a bit harder today because you took the push-up test first.

Even if the mountain climbers didn't seem harder, your push-ups probably will. Alternate doing one as fast as you can and then doing one as slowly as you can until you can't do any more.

Side planks today can combine the last two days by lifting both the top leg and reaching the top arm toward the ceiling. By doing this, we once again increase the balance challenge and thus increase the work load for our abs. As always, stay with an easier version if need be.

Lunge by stepping back today and you will further challenge your core. Alternate which leg you use to step back until you are fatigued.

Cool Down for Week One - Day Four

Cool down in the usual manner with low impact back kicks, reaching for the moon and lawn mowers. Now add the stretches we practiced yesterday. Start with the neck and work your way down.

Character Classics

We'll finish today's session by talking about our character classic, Tom Sawyer.
Talk about Mark Twain's notion that work is anything you feel obliged to do while play is anything you are

not obliged to do. Encourage personal examples as well as examples from the book. If time allows, listen to more of the story or also talk about Pollyanna or another book you have chosen to illustrate enthusiasm.

Character Challenge

See if there is a job or task to be done that you can turn into play with enthusiasm.

Mom's Moment

Take a minute to review the last few days and think of all the ways you saw family members trying to be enthusiastic. Tell them that you noticed. Give them a hug or two.

Week One - Day Five

It's time for a breakthrough workout. We'll push a little harder today. This will keep you from hitting a plateau and the challenge will be fun. With the weekend ahead, you're about to get a change of pace.

So attack today's workout with everything you've got.

Warm-Up for Week One - Day Five

In today's warm-up, we'll have some fun mixing up the various movements of the past four days. So everyone can choose whether they want to march, do straight leg kicks, kick to the side or kick to the back. Do a mix of all four if you like and only when you feel satisfied add the two dynamic stretches reaching for the moon and the lawn mower.

To Share with the Family

Warm and ready,, see if anyone can remember the definition of enthusiasm. See if anyone can spell it by standing on one foot and tracing the words in the air with the other foot. Be sure to do it twice so you can do it with the other leg. Feel free to use an easier word such as smile or fun.

Parent's Points to Ponder

Sometimes to understand a concept it helps to think about what it's opposite would be. The opposite of enthusiasm is dread or apathy. It has to do with expectations. Children expect Christmas or birthdays to be fun so they are filled with enthusiastic anticipation. Expect to have a good time every time you begin Exercising Values.

We have more control than we think so we should choose enthusiasm as a way of acknowledging that control. To never allow ourselves to be excited about something will protect us from disappointment, I suppose, but at what an enormous cost. Is anyone drawn to the apathetic person or the person who expects bad things to happen at every turn? Of course not. Allow yourself to be unabashedly enthusiastic about your family and the time you've set aside to spend with them. Remember the song, "shower the people you love with love, show them the way that you feel."

Breakthrough Workout for Week One - Day Five

In order for this to be a breakthrough workout you will need to take a short break and then do a second set of mountain climbers today.

For the push-up, vary the pace doing a 4/1 count, then a 2/2 count, then a 1/4 count. Next go as fast as you can followed by going as slowly as you can. You may be surprised to find that going slowly is actually harder than going fast.

Planks are a bit complex today but you will soon master this one. Begin as you did on day three with legs straight supporting yourself with the straight or bent arm. Your other arm is reaching overhead until you let it swing down between your body and the floor. Once again reach overhead. Continue to swing and reach until fatigue sets in. When it does, smoothly turn and change sides instead of swinging your arm between your body and the floor. This can be done once or change sides repeatedly to add more difficulty and to keep the exercise going.

Lunges can include all the variations you have learned so far. Step to the front or the back, do repeats with one leg at a time or lunge around the room. By switching off, you may be able to do more total lunges.

Cool Down for Week One - Day Five

Cool down should include a variety of movements just like the warm-up. Include your two dynamic stretches as well as the static stretches we learned yesterday. Partner stretches are a great way to finish this extra effort workout.

Character Classics

Even when you don't have time to listen to more of the story, you can mention the characters or ask questions about the plot and keep the story fresh in their minds. Build enthusiasm for the next time you will have the opportunity to listen to more of the story.

Character Challenge

Build some enthusiasm for tomorrow. Brain storm some active games you can do together for game day. Parents can teach a favorite game from their own childhood or as a family you could enjoy an activity that your kids love.

When I was a child, my mom taught me kick-the-can, a game she had played as a child. Soon twenty to thirty neighborhood children were gathering to play it over an area encompassing four houses each night. Seems strange to me now that not all of those houses even had children living there. Maybe neighborhoods were friendlier in those days or maybe we were just out of line.

So your plan for tomorrow might be to exercise together the old fashioned way or you might include a contemporary workout such as Wii Fit or laser tag. Just have fun. Mix it up.

Mom's Moment

Hopefully, thinking about some of the things you enjoyed as a child has stirred up some happy family memories. If so, is there anyone you could call today just to say hi and talk a few minutes? Maybe that would be your mom or dad, your grandmother or a sibling. If you don't have family maybe there is a neighbor or a friend that has been important in your life. Maybe there is even another family that you would like to invite to join you tomorrow for game day. See if you can take your enthusiasm for family and fitness and spread it around.

Saturday is Game Day

Today, we set aside the regular workout that during the week lasts twenty minutes or less. Instead, we will enjoy some extended time with our family. Use the ideas you thought of yesterday. Other suggestions could include frisbee on the beach or playing in the snow. You could go on a nature walk or play a game of tag in the back yard. Perhaps one of your children is in an organized sport and the family can turn out to support them. You could shoot a few baskets or hit a few tennis balls.

Just let today be active and fun and spend some of it together as a family. Later you may want to listen again to the excerpt from Tom Sawyer, begin listening to the entire book, or listen to Pollyanna. Story time may also be a good activity for tomorrow.

Sunday is Rest Day

One day a week should be a break from organized physical activity. This week you made a lot of changes and you need a break to absorb all the benefits. You may be experiencing metabolic fatigue from your multiple training sessions. You may have some tissue damage from the jumping and overall work loads. Your nervous system has tried some new activities and also deserves a rest.

Psychologically you may even be a bit stressed simply because you tried some new ways of relating to people or because you spent more time with your family. Yes, even happy events can cause stress. It is best to acknowledge that you need a break. Lifestyle issues unrelated to this program may be your greatest source of stress and it is good to just take some time to relax.

Mom's Moment

How about a nap? If you are hesitant consider this: getting behind on sleep is associated with the following:

1. Increased appetite and associated weight gain.

Do I really need a number two? Here it is anyway:

2. Impaired motor function and reaction time as well as delayed visual and auditory reaction time. If you drive your kids, enough said.

3. Impaired ability to replace the glycogen in your muscles leading to earlier fatigue in subsequent workouts.

4. Reduced cardiovascular performance.

5. Increased perceived exertion during workouts or strenuous routine activities.

6. Reduced motivation and impaired mood.

7. Reduced short-term memory.

Like I said, how about a nap? I hope you are enthusiastic about the idea.

Week Two - Day One

If I say the words strength training, do you immediately visualize barbells, dumbbells or the large pieces of equipment you'd find in a gym? The truth is, you have already been doing strength training utilizing just your body weight. You have been doing the kind that will help you shed weight and reveal lean muscles.

I am providing you with a total body exercise routine but that doesn't mean that you can't spend a little extra time on areas you consider weaknesses. If it's your legs, then really work those dead lifts this week. Even feel free to throw in a few lunges from last week. Or if it's your abs that concern you, realize that the full body exercises like burpees and mountain climbers will do more to burn the fat around the middle than endless crunches. That said, there is value in crunches and we will do a few this week.

Warm-Up for Week Two - Day One

Since we will be introducing four new exercises to this week's routines, we will keep the warm-ups and cool downs the same. I'll leave it up to you and your children to choose which movements you include. You can make a game of it and let each person call out march, front kick, sidekick, back kick, or free choice. This participation and ability to choose may make this one of your children's favorite parts of the exercise routine. Don't forget to include the reach for the moon and lawn mower. Next week, we will learn a whole new warm-up so enjoy this one while it lasts.

Before we begin the main workout, let's introduce the new character quality. Don't underestimate the value of having this new focus twirling in their heads while they are working out. Not only will they associate learning character with fun; they will also be more likely to retain new information.

Introducing the Character Quality

LOYALTY

Loyalty is demonstrating faithfulness and commitment even when it is difficult, inconvenient or even dangerous to do so.

To Share with the Family

Everyone loves the friend they can count on, the one who will stand by them no matter what. People respect the fire fighter who is loyal to community safety and will put his own life at risk to save others. Soldiers similarly deserve our respect because of their loyal sacrifices. We need to chose carefully what or to whom we are loyal, being sure they are worthy of our respect and trust.

Parent's Points to Ponder

How you spend your time certainly speaks to your loyalty to your family's welfare. Children understand the need for work but they are also sensitive to what you truly love. By setting aside the time for Exercising Values each and every day, you are speaking volumes about who and what is important to you. It's impossible to inspire loyalty without practicing it yourself. Stay rock solid in your loyal commitment to spending fun and meaningful time with your family. Dads should definitely be a part of this family program.

Workout for Week Two - Day One

Now let's learn some new exercises:

Let's get our heart rates up with burpees. Start in a front plank position, with feet as wide as your hip bones. Jump your feet in toward your hands by bending your knees and springing forward. You will land in a low squat. Now jump straight up as you reach high over head with your arms. As your feet touch down, you return to the squat and then immediately jump back into the plank with a straight back. Repeat several times to work your heart and lungs, chest, shoulders, abs, quads, glutes and calves.

Dips can be done from the floor, a piece of furniture or a stair. This will work your triceps, anterior deltoid and chest. Position your hands with fingers facing forward next to your side on the floor or on one of the objects just mentioned.

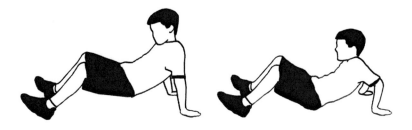

Lift your hips and support your lower body by pressing your feet into the floor. Keep your elbows close to your body. Lower your body as far as ninety degrees or what you are able to do while you inhale. Push-up with force exhaling as you do. Continue until fatigued and then move on to crunches.

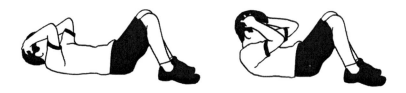

Crunch: Lie on your back with your knees bent and your feet flat on the floor. Place your hands behind your head but do not lace your fingers together. Elbows are out and should stay out. Do not tuck your chin. Take a deep breath in and as you exhale initiate curling up by contracting and activating your abdominal muscles. Pull your belly button toward your spine. Keep your chin up. Do not throw yourself up or tug on your neck or head. Your shoulder blades should rise a few inches and you'll return back down with control. Repeat as long as you are able to keep good form and avoid pausing.

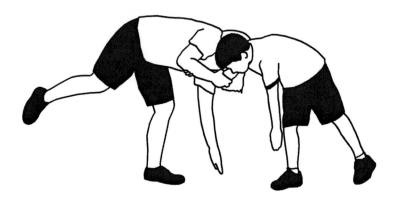

Partner One-Leg Dead Lifts: Now we'll finish by working the glutes, hamstrings and lower back. We will need to partner up for this one. Stand facing your partner and then each of you take a step to the right positioning yourselves so you can clasp your inside arms and be free to reach down with your outside arms. Begin with your feet slightly narrower than the width of your hip bones with your knees only slightly bent. Raise the outside foot up in the air as you reach below your knee with the outside arm. By clasping arms you have someone to steady you and yet you will challenge your own core when you in turn steady them. Repeat several times and then change arms.

As you progress, you may be able to just hold hands. If you do this advanced version, be aware that you are more likely to pull each other off balance.

Cool Down for Week Two - Day One

Cool down using the exercises from the warm-up. Once again, let the children call out which of the movements they want to do. These include marching and various kicks. Add the static stretch routine you learned on day three last week to your dynamic stretches: then reach for the moon and do the lawn mower.

Character Classics

My favorite book in the third grade was Black Beauty by Anne Sewell. The teacher read a few pages of the book aloud to the class each day. Our concern for this horse grew more intense each day as he faced various trials and hardships. I believe that your children will be moved by this classic much as I was so many years ago. After this book was read aloud to me, I read every book about horses that I could get my hands on. Being read to creates good readers.

It will help our children explore the concept of loyalty as they picture Black Beauty being passed from owner to owner. Having to form the images in their minds will stimulate their imaginations. You can ask questions to help them create detailed accounts in their minds and further stimulate their thinking.

If you have a pet, you might also talk about the loyalty between the members of your family and that pet. We have a golden retriever, a cocker spaniel mix and until his recent death, we also had a chocolate lab. All of our dogs have been protective and have exuded loyalty. Teaching children to responsibly care for a pet is a big step toward their maturity.

Character Challenge

Remind everyone that participating everyday with a good attitude is a great way to show their loyalty to the other family members. You are in this together. When you prioritize this family time, you are loyally helping everyone in the family be successful. Encourage each other by noticing improvements and good attitudes.

Studies show that people who work out with other people get better results than those who workout alone. Each family member is critical to the other members' success. A four year old who reminds his mom that it's time for Exercising Values could be the difference in whether that mom sticks with the program or gives up. Everyone's consistent participation is so valuable to the family.

Mom's Moment

Get a large glass of water and as you sip on it consider what you are going to do about the food in your house. Let's face it, soft drinks, candy, chips, and other packaged foods don't storm your house. You bring them in. What would it feel like to clean out the refrigerator and cabinets and replace junk foods with nutrient rich foods?

If you need help with food selections beyond those contained in this book you can also find a list of colleagues who specialize in nutrition that I personally recommend at www.exercisingvalues.com. Most of them will offer you free samples so you can judge for yourself if their information will be useful to your family.

Week Two - Day Two

Warm-Up for Week Two - Day Two

If the children are still enjoying calling out the warm-up exercises, then let them. If not, it can be the parents' chance to call the shots. Just remember to progress from small movements to larger movements and from low impact to ballistic movements. Let your bodies warm-up gradually.

To Share with the Family

Thank your children for the enthusiasm and loyalty they demonstrated during the warm-up. Remind them of the definition of loyalty: Loyalty is demonstrating faithfulness and commitment even when it is difficult, inconvenient or even dangerous to do so. Talk about why we need to wisely choose our friends and then commit to their well-being by staying loyal through good times and bad. A fair-weather friend isn't really a friend at all.

Parent's Points to Ponder

Loyalty is at the heart of the marriage commitment and observing children will note how their parents respond to each other. We always teach more by what we do and don't do than by what we say. I am not writing to the non-existent perfect, happy little family.

We all face real struggles, disappointments, and conflicts.

Not all conflicts are even resolvable. Sometimes they just need to be acknowledged and managed. Hurts have to be let go of so life can go on. Through all of this, a determination to remain loyal to your beliefs and highest values will protect you from compromises and make you more likely to be there for each other.

Workout for Week Two - Day Two

Go at your own pace and encourage everyone else in the family to do so, too. We add variations each day for variety and to keep you challenged. It is fine to stay at an easier level as long as it is working for you. Day by day, your abilities will increase and you'll be stronger.

Don't worry if you feel best staying at the same level for a long time. But don't let that stop you from acknowledging someone else's improvement. Strive to be a source of loyal, enthusiastic support for those around you. People vary in how quickly they adapt to exercise.

Burpee: Today when you shoot your legs out add a straddle with a quick jump back in.

Dip: Progress with your dips by stepping your feet further from your body or if you started on the floor progress to using a chair or a couple of stairs so you can go a bit deeper on the dip. If this bothers your shoulder, return to the floor version until you build more strength.

Crunch: Start your crunch at the top so rather than getting a momentary break at the bottom of each repetition you will need to contract hard as you pause at the top instead. This small change alone will dramatically increase the effectiveness of your crunches. Time under tension develops a muscle and this will keep tension on the muscle for a longer time.

Partner One-Leg Deadlifts: Lighten your grip or hold on further down your partner's arm. If your partner suddenly holds on tighter, you'll have to work your own core harder to avoid losing your balance. Be a team and help and encourage each other.

Cool Down for Week Two - Day Two

Do our routine cool down and stretch. This is another chance for everyone to call out their favorite movement. Include one or both partner stretches at the end, if you have time.

Character Classics

Because of the intensity of the story, you may find it is best absorbed in small doses. Although I expect your children will want to hear more. These recordings can be downloaded to a MP3 player but listening together is half the fun. Children will listen to a story they enjoy again and again and having the story recorded allows them to do this.

Character Challenge

Everyone should think of one of the things we have talked about previously that they could improve or take action on and then do it today. Grab that glass of water, make that phone call, give someone a hug or just go to bed earlier. The important thing is don't be forever learning and never doing. Do it.

Mom's Moment

Is there something left undone that weighs on you? If so, lessen the stress by just taking some action on it right now or at least sometime today. Take it's power to worry you away by proving you will get it done. Just like with exercise, a little consistent progress will add up and you'll be rewarded.

Week Two - Day Three

It's mid-week and we are settled into our routine. The new exercises should be familiar by now but still challenging. The concept of loyalty should be penetrating our hearts and minds.

Warm-Up for Week Two - Day Three

Warm-up as usual. Children will enjoy a sense of mastery and knowing what to expect.

To Share with the Family

Hard times provide opportunities to display loyalty. Rather than a self-centered complaining demeanor a person can rise to the occasion with encouraging words and acts of service. Loyal people refuse to criticize others but look for the good and the praiseworthy. Showing respect for others will teach your children not to mock or make fun of others.

Parent's Points to Ponder

Tho opposite of loyalty is betrayal. Loyalty comes out of gratitude for the past as well as belief in the future. It comes from a sense of belonging and being a part of something. To that extent it may not be deserved. Even abused children will exhibit loyalty to their parents. In a way, it is a twisted part of self-preservation because their identity is involved.

They'll chose emotional congruence over physical safety. As always, the value of loyalty is tied directly to the worthiness of what we have attached our loyalty to.

Workout for Week Two - Day Three

Burpee: Add a second leap into the air. When you land immediately spring back and try to jump even higher the second time. Then squat down and thrust your legs behind you. You can still add yesterday's straddle or just omit it today. Repeat several times.

Dip: Progress as you did yesterday.

Crunch: Start at the top again and descend slowly to a count of three and then spring up explosively on one count. Watch your head and neck and concentrate on your abs.

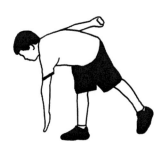

One-Leg Dead Lift: Let go of your partner and do these on your own. Be sure to switch sides. You'll continue to work your abs while working your hamstrings and back. You are developing proprioception or the sense of your body in space.

Cool Down for Week Two - Day Three

Cool down and stretch as usual.

Exercise Tips

Notice which exercises you struggle with the most. Next time concentrate on these by doing an extra set or a few extra reps. Identifying areas of weakness isn't enough. We need to work on them.

Character Classics

Look for examples of loyalty as you listen to the story today.

Character Challenge

Practice loyalty by pointing out the good in others today. If you look hard enough you'll see what others are doing right. Tell them so.

Mom's Moment

Take a moment to identify what is starting to come a bit easier to you. Reflect on your strengths and those of others in the family. Encourage yourself with these thoughts and turn your positive observations of others into words and let them know. If you hope that your children will respond to today's challenge be sure that you are leading by example. All of us, but especially children, learn best from those who demonstrate genuine love and true concern.

Week Two - Day Four

According to the National Weight Loss Registry 78% of those who keep off thirty pounds or more for at least a year eat breakfast regularly. Therefore, 22% did not. So it can be done. I know you probably expected me to say that it means you should eat breakfast. It means you probably should eat breakfast. There are general rules and lots of exceptions and you need to notice the results you get from various actions.

Notice if eating breakfast curbs your appetite and sets you up for controlled healthy eating all day. Notice if skipping breakfast leaves you moody, with low energy or causes you to binge on whatever you find later in the day. Of course, all breakfasts aren't equal so your investigation will need to continue until you find which balance of protein, fats, carbs and calories make you feel best. Factor in convenience and affordability and voila you didn't really need me or anyone else to tell you what or when to eat in the morning.

Now, of course, go feed the kids. We'll just assume they'll feel and learn better when they eat the nutritious meal you have in mind. If you do Exercising Values in the morning, they may be more motivated to eat a healthy breakfast. It puts all of us in better touch with the nutrition needs of our bodies.

Warm-Up for Week Two - Day Four

Warm-up as usual. Be sure everyone has a chance to choose which movement to do next. This method will keep some variety in your warm-up while still using movements with which you are familiar.

To Share with the Family

Taking care of people as they age is an important part of loyalty and a way for us to show gratitude for all they've added to our lives. Consider the elderly people in your life and think of ways to show your loyalty to them.

Parent's Points to Ponder

At every stage and age of your children's lives, it is good to know their friends. Friends have a tremendous influence on our lives. Plus, you may be helpful even as a role model for one of their friends who might not get much attention at home.

Workout for Week Two - Day Four

Add a push-up to that burpee, Rocky. Yep, you are getting stronger. Maybe not strong enough to do Rocky style one-arm push-ups, but strong nevertheless.

Dips and more dips. Do your best.

Crunch from the top but reverse the count. This time go down on one count and up on three.

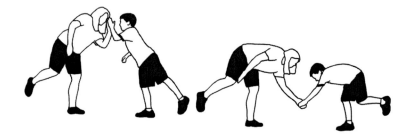

While doing your one-leg dead lifts see if you and your partner can high five then low five. See how hard you can clap without either of you losing your balance. Have some fun with this and be nice.

Cool Down for Week Two - Day Four

Cool down and stretch as usual.

Character Classics

Be sure to give your kids a chance to share their feelings about the story. Share with them your feelings, too. Let them ask you any questions that the story may have raised.
It's an emotional story that teaches a lot about life and loss.

Character Challenge

Widen your children's view about the world by sharing with them about children who need help getting food in order to survive. You could take food to a local shelter or let the kids earn money to send overseas to an orphanage or other shelter. While we are trying to learn to not eat excessively ourselves, it is good to be involved in helping those who may not be able to eat at all today. Being loyal to the less fortunate is a cornerstone of good character.

Mom's Moment

Take time today to enjoy and really notice a healthy snack. Take time to reflect on what you and your kids habitually eat and make a plan for how you are going to improve it. Rethink your relationship with processed foods.

Good nutrition doesn't have to be hard but it does take a little fore thought. Avoid fast foods by planning head. If you had it available, what would you really like to eat and feed your kids today? Planning will get you your first choice instead of settling for whatever you can find quickly.

Week Two - Day Five

Warm-Up for Week Two - Day Five

Hopefully, today finds you healthy and ready for a more intense workout. Put a little extra oomph into your warm-up as we will be replacing it next week with an alternative warm-up. Really reach for the moon figuratively and literally.

To Share with the Family

Talk about loyalty to your country and teach them what this means to you. Let them know about any sacrifices anyone in your family or lineage has made for their country.
Keep it personal rather than a history lesson, although you should share about any aspect of your national heritage that has great meaning to you.

Parent's Points to Ponder

If someone just looked at how you spend your time, to what or to whom would they say you were most loyal? Is that the way you want it to be or do you need to make some changes so your time reflects what is truly important to you?

Breakthrough Workout for Week Two - Day Five

Burpees will have a lot of extras today. Add a straddle jump out and in, next add a push-up and finish with an extra jump up. Do a few more burpees than usual. This is your breakthrough day so do your very best.

Dips: If your hands are on a chair you can also elevate your feet onto another chair to increase the weight you are pushing up. Otherwise, just do more dips than usual to increase the difficulty. A ninety degree angle or less is all you need so don't drop too low.

Crunch: Start at the top and first do a set of 10 on a 3/1 count and then a set at a 1/3 count. Add a 2/2 count set and repeat all three as long as you can.

Dead Lift: When you change sides today keep your foot up until you've hopped into position. Do as many as you can on each side before changing sides and change sides until you are fatigued. Remember to keep your foot off the ground as long as you can.

Cool Down for Week Two - Day Five

Cool down and stretch as usual.

Character Classics

Classics are meant to be enjoyed again so keep a copy when you finish the novel. Someone in the family may want to spend more time with it.

Character Challenge

Be especially kind and loyal to your brothers and sisters today. Think of something you could do to make game day tomorrow more fun for them.

Mom's Moment

Do something you love to do today. Just do it.

Saturday is Game Day

You know what to do. Have fun. Make a big deal out of it. Make it memorable.

Sunday is Rest Day

Taking a break from organized physical activity doesn't mean you have to stay on the couch. Just do what relaxes and refreshes you. Maybe a walk outside, a movie, or a game. Everyone needs some discretionary time in their lives.

Week Three - Day One

Congratulations on making it to week three! You are well on your way to developing the life long habit of daily exercise. You have invested in your children and they will always remember this demonstration of your love and commitment. I hope the improvements you see in your energy and appearance help you realize that you can control how you look and feel through consistent daily action.

Warm-Up for Week Three - Day One

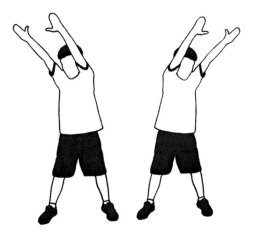

Can it be any simpler? We are going to warm-up by running in place, running outside or running around the room. Next, leap from side to side. Stop and wave your arms overhead back and forth.

In a wide straddle, do a dynamic stretch by shifting your weight side to side. Repeat each of these until your heart rate is up a bit and you feel warm.

Introducing the Character Quality

DILIGENCE

Diligence is the steady application of effort to accomplish a task. Though we associate it with hard work it is actually derived from a Latin word, diligo, which means earnest love. If you love what you do and do it on behalf of those you love; diligence will naturally follow. The opposite of being diligent is being lazy or half-hearted in what you undertake. Let's be diligent with the new workout.

To Share with the Family

As much as we try to keep the fun in what we do, we all know that it is necessary to keep going even when something seems tedious or dull. The ability to stick with something until it is completed is very valuable. Concentrating when it would be easier to allow yourself to be distracted is admirable. In fact, the ability to concentrate is even associated with genius. Taking care to follow instructions and do a job right helps us get good results and the resulting satisfaction.

Parent's Points to Ponder

Strive to demonstrate diligence with your own exercise program. Exercising Values isn't something we just do for the kids because it is good for them. It is also good for you. Be excited about your own successes and progress. Allow your children to see you sweat as you put forth the effort to get an extra squat or pull-up. Don't quit when it isn't easy and they won't quit either.

Workout for Week Three - Day One

Jumping Jacks: Parents may need to teach this familiar movement to their children. Be patient remembering that as long as arms are moving and legs are jumping, then bodies are being benefitted.

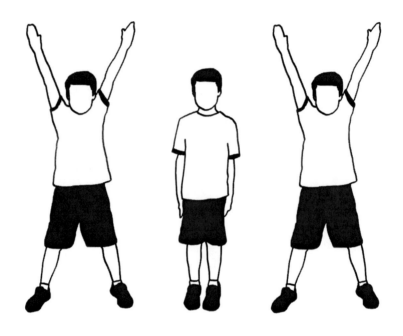

Running Arms: Just like it sounds, we are going to vigorously move the arms back and forth in the running motion. If you drive the arm back it will naturally swing back to the front. Keep the arms up rather than out and keep the hands close to the face.

Team Pull-Ups: Partners need to be close to the same size or alternatively parents can always be the standing partner. The standing partner gets considerable core work from their end of the exercise so if at all possible it is best to have a turn as the standing partner as well as the partner on the floor.

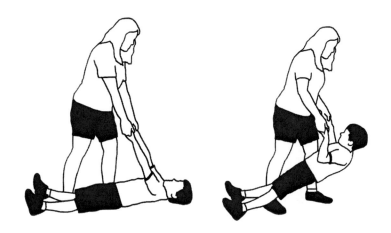

One person lies on their back and reaches their arms up to clasp the arms of their partner who is straddling them and reaching their arms down toward them. The standing person braces themselves by tightening their abs and moving their feet until they feel secure. This person does not pull the other person up. They just offer their arms for the lying person to use to pull themselves up after first tightening their core.

This person will then lower themselves down. Repeat a few times and then change places if you can. If there is no one available, you can also stand leaning back in a doorway and pull yourself to an upright position by pulling on the door frame. It lacks the camaraderie of the partner set up but it will get the job done.

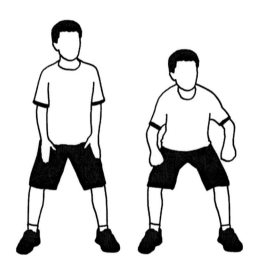

Squat: You get the whole package with this one; working the glutes, hamstrings and quads, Stand with your feet as wide as your hip bones. Keep your weight slightly more on your heels. Square your shoulders and tighten your abs. Look straight ahead or slightly up.

Sit back as though sitting into a low chair. Alternatively, think of it as sitting back onto a high stool, if getting as low as 90 degrees is too difficult or uncomfortable. Someone in the family can watch to be sure your knees stay behind your toes. They can even place their hand directly above your toes so if you hit it with your knee you'll know you should go no further. Don't arch your back or bend forward. Instead, keep the back straight as you lower and rise again.

Cool Down for Week Three - Day One

After squatting, you won't need to run or leap side to side. Instead, alternate lifting each leg high and hug them to your chest several times. Wave your arms. Straddle and shift your weight side to side. Do the stretches we learned in the previous weeks.

Character Classics

Louisa May Alcott's story, Little Men, will be our vehicle for discussing diligence. The diligence of the boys as well as those who care for them will shine through in this warm-hearted novel.

Character Challenge

Diligently complete a task you have been putting off. Try to make it something that will truly make your life better or easier. Sorry kids, but cleaning your room would fit that description. But then again the diligent parent sometimes takes their kids to the zoo.

You work it out. Whatever you decide, try to do it with enthusiasm. Taking care of responsibilities is one way to be loyal. Good character qualities always overlap so continue to reinforce the ones we have previously learned.

Exercise Tips: When we do the partner pull-ups, you'll have a chance to practice team work and to build each other up. Don't miss this opportunity.

Mom's Moment

By the end of this week you will have put in the 21 days that some researchers say it takes to form a new habit. Never mind that other researchers say it is more like 40-60 days, The important thing is everyday you are improving your children's lives by investing time in their fitness, health and character. Think about any positive changes you have noticed and let that be your incentive for pressing on.

Week Three - Day Two

Warm-Up for Week Three - Day Two

We are once again going to warm-up by running in place, running outside or running around the room. Then, it's time to leap from side to side. Next, wave your arms overhead back and forth. In a wide straddle do a dynamic stretch by shifting your weight side to side. Repeat each of these until your heart rate is up a bit and you feel warm.

To Share with the Family

The opposite of diligence is laziness. It is refusing to be focused, disciplined, and to apply oneself to a task. It is quitting too soon and not seeing something through. No one wants to pass on laziness to their children. Strive to be diligent so they can model themselves off of you.

Parent's Points to Ponder

I never felt like I had a blank slate with my children. Rather, they seemed to come with a purpose. I'll never forget that steely blue gaze from Jennifer, my first-born, the first time we locked eyes. To me, she seemed to be a person to be discovered.

That said, we will never have more influence for good or for bad as we do with our own children. It is an awesome responsibility that occurs in so many unplanned moments. It always surprises me when one of my kids recalls something we did or something I said that I have completely forgotten.

Trying to bring out the best in someone else requires us to diligently try to be the best we can be. No child is impressed with "do as I say not as I do" although it could work for a while. People, especially children, want to be inspired. They want someone to look up to. Look at the dubious characters within the media vying to be that person your child admires. Wouldn't you rather hold that coveted position yourself?

Workout for Week Three - Day Two

It's time once again to exercise together, We are going to repeat the workout from day one. Jumping jacks and squats are such basic movement that they need to be mastered. Many trainers say if they could only do one exercise it would be the squat. There are many variations to keep this basic exercise fresh.

Running arms will lay the foundation for efficient running. In running, the arms control the legs. It is good to learn how to run with a quiet upper body and relaxed arms. They should be in close to the body and bent at ninety degrees or a bit more.

Partner pull-ups should make these sessions fun and you'll have a chance to practice team work and to build each other up. Don't miss this opportunity. Pair off in ways that allow everyone to have a good experience.

These exercises can be returned to time and again when you need a quick effective workout. Remember this when you are traveling and the hotel doesn't have a gym. You'll never again be able to use that as an excuse to miss a workout. Keep it simple.

Cool Down for Week Three - Day Two

Alternate lifting each leg high and hug them to your chest several times. Begin quickly and then slow down as you go. Move on to waving your arms. Straddle and shift your weight side to side. Do the stretches we learned in the previous weeks. Include some partner stretches if you like.

Character Classics

Talk about the boys' lives and how they are different or are the same as your lives.

Character Challenge

We will continue each day to apply diligence to something that you would love to mark off your to do list. Children will learn the benefit of getting things done. Whether you finish one big project or several small ones, revel in your new found freedom.

Parents, don't forget to diligently provide a special outing that requires extra effort on your part, even if it's just a trip to the park or library. Your children will learn first hand that diligent people make things better and more interesting for others.

Mom's Moment

Now that you've successfully established a healthy habit take the next few days to create a list of other habits you'd like to establish. Take them on one or two at a time. You have proven to yourself that you can create good changes in your life. Mimic what you have already done with Exercising Values to create action steps for other changes you'd like to make. Start small but take consistent daily action.

Week Three - Day Three

Warm-Up for Week Three - Day Three

Run, leap, wave and straddle. This is a repeat of yesterday's warm-up.

To Share with the Family

Mastering a skill takes diligent practice. Think of all the things you are trying to learn and try to apply diligence to your efforts. It comes down to doing your best with a little zest. The combination of enthusiasm and diligence will allow you to accomplish more than just resigning yourself to a task. Attitude is so important, so do all you can to choose one that will get you where you need to go.

Discuss the notion of what it means to be a hard worker. Talk about doing a good job even when no else is watching. Introduce the concept of finding satisfaction in a job well-done.

Parent's Points to Ponder

Children are born to move. That means you are meant to move, too. Exercising Values is playful. You should chose to smile and at times it will make you laugh. As you rediscover this natural bent toward being active, you will begin to own this program and your transformation. The effects of months or years of inactivity will melt away and you will feel more alive.

Do you really want the image your children have of you to be you tucked up on the sofa with a bag of chips and a cool one? Really? Or do you want them to remember you laughing, playing, and teaching? Let the routine of Exercising Values cement your legacy as someone who really cared about them.

Workout for Week Three - Day Three

Jumping jacks are probably getting easier and your running arms feel more natural. By now everyone has either found a good partner for the pull-ups or is making due in a doorway. In future months, we will build on the squats that you are doing now by adding overhead movements and by doing one-leg squats. For now, it is important to master this basic exercise that you will use daily throughout life.

Cool Down for Week Three - Day Three

Once again, alternate lifting each leg high and hug them to your chest several times. Begin quickly and then slow down as you go. Move on to waving your arms. Straddle and shift your weight side to side. Repeat each of these until you are ready to do the stretches we learned in the previous weeks.

Character Classics

Little Men was based on Louisa May Alcott's own experiences. Talk about acknowledging anyone in your family that has an interesting story to tell from their life. Children love to hear stories from their parent's childhood and this would be a great time to tell one.

Character Challenge

Diligence isn't just about doing. We can also be diligent in the way we apply ourselves to things like listening and understanding. How well did you listen while others told their stories today? Did you try to understand their point of view? See how well you can listen to others today.

Mom's Moment

Listening is especially important for a mother. We need to listen to our own hearts as well as to all the people who need our attention. Sometimes it is so overwhelming that you need to find a few moments of silence just to re-charge. If today is one of those days, try to find just a few moments of solitude, even if it is only just before sleep tonight.

Week Three - Day Four

Warm-Up for Week Three - Day Four

It's the basics again today. Begin by running in place or all about. Change the order and wave your arms next. As your heart starts to slow down, switch to leaps and then finish with your straddle stretch.

To Share with the Family

When Olympic winners or other successful athletes are interviewed they will often speak about the years of training that went into their achievement. Is there anything, whether it be sports, music, charity work, academic studies or anything else, that you love so much that you can see yourself dedicating years to work to perfect it? If anyone in the family has such a dream, this would be an opportunity to share it.

Parent's Points to Ponder

Dreams aren't just for the young ones. Share your hopes and dreams with each other or with a close friend. If you commit to pursuing them diligently, you could achieve them. Reflect on any dreams you'd like to pursue. Then hold onto that dream.

Workout for Week Three - Day Four

Let's do the workout in reverse order from yesterday. Begin with squats and then do partner pull-ups. Running arms are next and then conclude with jumping jacks. Repeat this one to three more times.

Cool Down for Week Three - Day Four

Begin by waving your arms but then quickly move to lifting each leg and hugging it to your chest several times. Straddle and shift your weight side to side. Repeat each of these until you are ready to do the stretches from the top down beginning with the neck.

Character Classics

Is there an act of service in the book that you could emulate?

Character Challenge

If someone wrote a book about your life what acts of service would there be for someone to emulate?

Mom's Moment

While we are on the subject of emulation, take a moment to think of any area of your life that you hope your children won't copy. If so, is there anything you can do to change that area of your life. If not, reflect on how you will lead them a different direction. Is it something that you will feel better about if you talk to them about it?

Week Three - Day Five

Warm-Up for Week Three - Day Five

A thorough warm-up is particularly important today because we will be adding some intensity. Warm-up by running in place, running outside or running around the room followed by leaping from side to side. Today, you might want to add skipping or galloping.

Young children may need some time and practice to learn these movements but they'll enjoy the variety and challenge. Adults may feel silly at first skipping but let me assure you that elite running coaches often include drills like skipping in their programs for top notch athletes. Besides, your kids will love it when you join in and you may feel like a kid yourself.

Don't forget to wave your arms overhead back and forth to warm up the upper body. In a wide straddle do a dynamic stretch by shifting your weight side to side. Repeat each of these until your heart rate is up a bit and you feel warm.

To Share with the Family

The exercise routines are simple but they are backed by research and lots of experience. They will get you fit. Watch your diet and they will get you lean and fit. The greatest body in the world is worthless if the soul within it is wanting. Character trains actions but it also trains mood, attitude, and ensures joy, if not happiness. Diligence in teaching character now will reap great rewards later.

Parent's Points to Ponder

Being active with you provides your children a hedge against the many things that may discourage activity later like being picked last in gym class, injury, or even busyness. People gravitate back to activities that created fond memories. Some of what you eat is probably dictated by an association with a happy or relaxing memory. Decide to diligently work to create happy memories linked to health, fun, and family.

Breakthrough Workout for Week Three - Day Five

The breakthrough day is back and you now have more strength and stamina to apply to your special efforts. We'll stay with jumping jacks, running arms, partner pull-ups and squats but increase the sets and reps. Be happy with your progress and enjoy the sensation that your cardiovascular system is getting stronger so you can work longer and harder without needing to rest. Congratulate yourself for growing yourself this far and for leading your family.

Cool Down for Week Three - Day Five

Stick with the cool down you have been doing. Alternate lifting each leg high and hug them to your chest several times. Begin quickly and then slow down as you go. Move on to waving your arms. Straddle and shift your weight side to side. Do the stretches we learned in the previous weeks. Conclude with some partner stretches.

Character Classics

This might be a great time just to let your children know that you are glad they are in your family. Ask them what they learned about the importance of family from Little Men.

Character Challenge

Let the whole family in on the mom's moment and let everyone try to think of something special to do for someone else in the family. If you have a large family and don't want anyone to be left out you could even draw names and do the kindness secretly.

Mom's Moment

Let's balance the extra effort you put into your workout with taking a day off from all those projects. Life is all about balance. Use the extra time to do something special for someone in the family just for the fun of it.

Saturday is Game Day

With so many things marked off your to do list, you should feel more relaxed and ready to play. Help make the connection between diligent work and well-deserved play time. Teach the balanced lifestyle that includes work and play. Today... PLAY!

Sunday is Rest Day

This may be a good day to listen to this week's character classic. It's a day set aside for rest and renewal, however you define that.

Mom's Moment

Repeat the exercise we did on day one. Relax with your eyes closed and visualize the benefits you hope your family will receive from this program. Imagine it in detail. Note the progress you are making. Take a deep breath and smile. You are doing the best you can for your kids.

Week Four - Day One

It may surprise you to learn that elite athletes don't train in a linear fashion with each week always more challenging than the week before. Instead periodically, often every fourth week, they will take a step back to fully recover and consolidate gains. We are already using one full day each week for rest. Many people find it hard to go longer than three weeks of increasing work loads before they need an easy week. This is that easy week. Recovery times increase with age so this will help the parents keep up with the children.

I want you to purposely do fewer reps and sets. Easy does it. We'll do enough to maintain our fitness while ensuring our complete recovery. This will feel similar to a taper in sports where volume is reduced but intensity is maintained. That way we can treat day 6 as a big event. You will be rested and ready to take on a more elaborate game day.

Warm-Up for Week Four - Day One

Warm-up is an opportunity to revisit the first three weeks. Today, we'll return to week one day one. You'll remember that we begin with a march but keep your feet close to the floor and your arms by your side. Next advance to a regular march and move your arms as well. Finally do an exaggerated march with your arms swinging high into the air. Now do all three sizes again but this time add a little bounce to your movements.

You have spent the past three weeks figuratively reaching for the moon. As you put one foot in front of the other and rock back and forth, reach high to remind you that you are on the road to success. As you pull back your prize by bringing both elbows in and back, realize that you can claim the health and fitness you desire. Do this several times. Change which foot is in front and repeat.

It's time to start that lawn mower. Stand with your feet apart in a straddle. Now bend and reach to one side by the floor and past your foot. Pull back and up. Repeat a few times and then change sides and do it all again.

Introducing the Character Quality

HOSPITALITY

Hospitality is sharing what you have with others.

To Share with the Family

Although we associate hospitality with welcoming someone into our homes for a meal or to spend the night, there are smaller acts of hospitality available all the time. The simple act of giving up your seat or warmly introducing a new person to your other friends are acts of hospitality. It is making others feel welcomed, wanted, and cared for. It is looking after their practical needs as well as making them feel at home.

The opposite of hospitality is stinginess. Hospitality is all about sharing and considering someone else as more important. Some cultures so esteem the stranger that Americans are astounded by the generosity of the poorest people. They will only give their very best to strangers no matter the cost. They inspire the rest of us to be less selfish.

Parent's Points to Ponder

Hospitality fights loneliness in yourself and others. While you want to open your home to others, you also want to be sure that all those living in your home feel like an important part of the family. Look for signs of loneliness in the people in your own family and be sensitive to their need to talk or spend time with you. A habitual welcoming smile lets everyone know that you are interested in them and approachable.

Welcome your children into your life. Practice this form of hospitality with them. Light up when you see them. Let them know you are glad to see them. Be ready to share your life lessons with them, to mentor them, and guide them.

Exercising Values is here to strengthen your resolve to protect your children's environment and to help you be successful in raising happy, healthy children who are bonded to you because they see how much you love them on a daily basis. Don't trade this great opportunity to make a difference in their lives by getting too busy with less important things. Build the character qualities into their lives a little at a time each day and like a tiny mustard seed it will yield much more than what you planted.

Workout for Week Four - Day One

Easy does it as we repeat workouts from each of the previous weeks. Today we'll return to week one and do mountain climbers, push-ups, side planks, and lunges. See if they come a bit easier now than they did that first workout.

Celebrate your progress but don't overdo it. Remember we are cutting back just a bit. The exciting thing is that what is a reduced workout today may still be more than you were able to do just a few short weeks ago. You are a champion!

Cool Down for Week Four - Day One

Let's take our cool down from a different week. Try this from week three: alternate lifting each leg high and hug them to your chest several times. Begin quickly and then slow down as you go. Move on to waving your arms. Straddle and shift your weight side to side. Do the top down stretch routine and finish with some partner stretches.

Character Classics

Same author but this time the book is Little Women. Enjoy the story of how the March sisters share their Christmas with a needing family and in the process make their own even more special. Noticing the differences in the four sisters might spur a conversation about the uniqueness of everyone in your family.

Character Challenge

Go through your things and see if there are things that are in good condition that you no longer need and could pass on to someone in need. Add at least one thing that is new and give it to a local shelter or charity. I have never forgotten the look of delight a boy at a shelter got at a Christmas party when he received a pencil. Yes, you read that right, a pencil. Sometimes we just can't imagine what others do without while we take those same things for granted.

Mom's Moment

Each day think of something nice to do for each member of your family including yourself and do it. It doesn't have to be something big, just something to help you connect.

Week Four - Day Two

Warm-Up for Week Four - Day Two

Simplicity today will give even our minds a break. So we are returning to week three day one in which we warm-up by running in place, running outside or running around the room. Next leap from side to side and put some joy into it. Keep up that enthusiasm as you switch to waving your arms overhead. In a wide straddle, do a dynamic stretch by shifting your weight side to side. Your inner thighs will love this one. Repeat each of these until your heart rate is up a bit and you feel warm.

To Share with the Family

Make these character qualities a part of the fiber of your being. We associate humility with Abe Lincoln and compassion with Mother Teresa. There will be a character quality or it's opposite that you will be known for and remembered. It will be your signature trait. Take care. Try them all on. Take your time. Let your children take their time.

Parent's Points to Ponder

A good coach sees what even an elite athlete can't see. Get a big picture and be a coach to your kids. Think about who has benefitted you in life. Trace the steps leading up to things you regret doing or not doing. Help someone with less life experience to build their life from what you already paid the price to learn. Be generous, supportive, and involved.

Walk closely with your children while they are young and they will be closer to you as they grow up. Children are very forgiving. They don't expect you to be perfect. They long for your love and acceptance. They particularly hope you accept that they aren't perfect either.

Workout for Week Four - Day Two

Week two day four was a bit harder with the added jump on the burpees so we will repeat it today with a bit of caution. Hopefully, it will seem easier to you now than it did two weeks ago. Have fun and enjoy your increased fitness but don't forget that this is a recovery week and your long term success will come quicker when you take time to rest. So cut back if it feels too hard. You will probably notice on the dead lifts that your balance has improved considerably. Here's a refresher on the workout:

Burpee: Add a second leap into the air. When you land immediately spring back and try to jump even higher the second time. Then squat down and thrust your legs behind you. You can still add yesterday's straddle if you feel very strong but otherwise just omit it today. Repeat several times but stop at a point where you know you could have done a few more.

Dip: Stop while it still seems easy. No need to push today.

Crunch: Start at the top again and descend slowly to a count of three and then spring up explosively on one count. Don't pull on your head and neck and concentrate on your abs. Contract hard at the top.

Dead Lift: Let go of your partner and do these on your own. Be sure to switch sides.

Cool Down for Week Four - Day Two

Cool down by lifting each leg high and hug them to your chest several times. Then we'll move right to a reversed order of our stretching routine. Start at the bottom and work up. This is the perfect day to give your flexibility a bit more focus. Take your time and enjoy each stretch.

These stretches should seem familiar but we will review them. Beginning with the lower body, use the wall or training partner to brace against. Placing one foot in front of the other, much like the beginning of a lunge, will allow you to lower the back heel towards the ground to stretch the calf. Then if you shift your weight back towards your back leg, you can lift the toes up and back on the front leg. By leaning over that leg you'll achieve a stretch for the hamstrings or back of the leg.

Holding on to the wall, a piece of furniture or your partner will allow you to then stretch the quads or front of the leg. This is done by bending your leg behind you and holding onto your ankle and gently pulling. When you release the leg, cross it behind the other leg and lean to each side for an IT band stretch. Repeat with the other leg.

To stretch the triceps bend your arm over your head and reach down your back. By placing the hand of your other arm just above the elbow of the stretching arm you may achieve a better stretch. Repeat on the other side.

Now take one arm across the body and assist the stretch with your other arm just above or below the elbow of the stretching arm. After holding this for 15-30 seconds look over the shoulder of the arm you are not stretching while still holding on to your arm. Now return to the front and drop your shoulder down as you still hold onto your arm. This pattern will stretch first the shoulder then the back. Next, it will stretch the shoulder again in a slightly different way. This should be repeated on the other side.

Now switch to a dynamic stretch by bring your arms out to the side and then alternate between rounding the arms and back as though you were hugging a big tree and drawing your arms back and pushing the chest out.

We'll finish with the neck. Take some extra time with this today and really try to relax. Stand straight with your arms at your sides. Reach towards the floor with your finger tips. Move your head to one side for a count of thirty and then move it to the other side.

Character Classics

Maybe there is someone you know who would really appreciate the thoughtfulness of receiving a meal from you. New mothers, the sick, and people who have just moved in would be some examples. Or alternatively, you could gather up some canned goods and drop them by a collection bin. In Little Women, the March family noticed when someone needed help and so should we. There is something very special about helping people who can't repay you. Don't think of hospitality as just having friends over. Reach out to people who need help as well.

Character Challenge

Try to purposely do something to demonstrate each of the four character qualities we have learned. Share what you've been up to with your family. Celebrate each others efforts.

Mom's Moment

It's okay to practice a bit of hospitality with yourself right now. Put your feet up, sip some ice water or tea and think about how your family life has improved these past few weeks.

Week Four - Day Three

Warm-Up for Week Four - Day Three

Warm-up by running in place, running outside or running around the room. Switch to skipping or galloping to add a little fun. Now wave your arms overhead back and forth to warm up the upper body. In a wide straddle, do a dynamic stretch by shifting your weight side to side. Repeat each of these until your heart rate is up a bit and you feel warm.

To Share with the Family

People who are new to an area are usually hoping to make new friends. Think together about anyone who is new to your neighborhood, church, school, work place, etc. and see if there is a way to include them in one of your family's activities. Also, just talk about the importance of smiling and being friendly to let new people know you are glad they are there.

Parent's Points to Ponder

As you progress through the fifty-two character qualities that make up a full years program, you will naturally gravitate toward seven or eight of them. Seven or eight will also seem less important to you but I can assure you that they might be the key seven or eight to someone else. Please try to consider each one and trust that it will be vital to your child's success and happiness.

As you begin to place more emphasis on a character quality that you have previously not deemed important, you may find relationships with others are improved. After all, when we value what someone else values it makes us closer. Allow the quality to settle.

Turn it around in your mind during the day, before you fall asleep, and when you wake up. Mull it over. Associate it with scripture or famous quotations you remember and are drawn to. Relax. There won't be a test. There may be life tests where your character shines through but that will come naturally.

Workout for Week Four - Day Three

Jumping jacks, running arms, partner pull-ups and squats will make up our routine today. I'd like you to do about half of what you think you can do of one and then move on to the next exercise. Continue circling through the workout until you've done each of them four or five times. We are stepping it up just a bit mid-week so this time you may feel a bit fatigued as you finish.

Cool Down for Week Four - Day Three

Use back kicks to bring your heart rate down. Reach for the moon. Finish by doing the total body stretching routine.

Character Classics

Little Women does have a death in the family and children may want to talk about this. Be prepared to teach them what you think they are ready to understand. Remind them that we want to make the most of every day we have with someone because they may exit our lives for any number of reasons. Today is the day you have to show love to the people in your life.

Character Challenge

If there is someone with whom you have had an argument or misunderstanding, today would be a great day to seek reconciliation.

Mom's Moment

Non-verbal communication is part of the way we tell people they are welcome or to stay away. Be sure your expressions and body language are sending the message you intend. Make it simple and go give your kids a hug.

Week Four - Day Four

Warm-Up for Week Four - Day Four

Straddle and lean side to side until you feel ready to leap. Take your leaps in a zig zag pattern. You have laid the ground work to handle this agility training. Practicing this now will help your child in many sports. Most children will have fun with this. Add a reach for the moon you should be ready to go.

To Share with the Family

What could be less hospitable than making fun of someone? Even when others are doing it, refuse to be a part of this cruel practice. Remember to treat other people the way you would want to be treated and mocking will simply not be a part of your life. Parents need to watch what they say about other people. Lead by example by refusing to gossip or speak unkindly.

Parent's Points to Ponder

Never turn on your children by using character to belittle or berate or to remind them that they fell short. Inspire don't bludgeon. What you think is reminding might be felt as discouraging or nagging. Be the hospitable host. Always be gracious and kind, especially with your children, who in fact, are guests in your home for a little while and then they move on. Value and use the time you have with them to help them on their way to a fulfilling life.

Studies say we should use five praises for every one criticism. I don't know. I think maybe just the five praises would do. Most of us are pretty good at knowing our own imperfections. If there is a blind spot you feel you must address, wait for the right moment.

I'm addressing self-concept. Parents are obliged to correct behavior. Still there is a balance. Hold to high standards for behavior but let them know no failure can separate them from your love. There is no need to hide your faults or to pretend to be better than they are. Love openly.

Let them see you working on your own character, failing, apologizing or seeking forgiveness when appropriate and then trying again. Don't even pretend to be above it all. Be the hungry beggar telling them where you found food not the pompous, self-satisfied know it all.

Be a student as well as a teacher. What you might get away with now will surely be tossed aside as adolescence sets in if you are not genuine, transparent, and obviously on their side. We don't own our children. They are with us for a time. Practice making them feel like a welcomed addition to your life and practicing hospitality with others will come that much easier.

Workout for Week Four - Day Four

We're going to mix it up today and start with dips, then squats, side planks, and then we'll hold a push-up after we lower down. Two times through should do it for this intense combination.

Cool Down for Week Four - Day Four

Alternate lifting each leg high and hug them to your chest several times. Straddle and shift your weight side to side. Move on to waving your arms. Then spend some time with this favorite partner stretch: one person is kneeling down with their bottom on their heels and they reach as far forward as they can while looking straight down at the floor. When they can't reach any further forward their partner will slowly and gently push first on the middle of their back and then on the top of their back to help their partner reach just a bit further. You can switch places and both of you will feel great.

By cutting back just a bit this week and by being very attentive to stretching we have set ourselves up for a great start to next month's program. I hope you feel relaxed and happy.

Character Classics

Settle in to this special family time. Some days you should just listen and enjoy the story as it unfolds and save the discussions for another time.

Character Challenge

See if everyone can name all four character qualities and their definitions. An example works just as well. Be sure to acknowledge it when you see these qualities in each other. The rest of the world may praise you for your looks or accomplishments but this goes much deeper and recognizes that you are becoming a person of substance.

Mom's Moment

You are so brave to be finding a way to help your children avoid a life time of problems. You are creative and expressive and loving. You have taken the right steps to help your family.

Relax. Let confidence overtake you and worries fall away. You are the mother you hoped to be and your children will remember how much you loved them and how hard you were willing to work to protect them. You pulled them out of the current when the culture wanted to hold them captive. You are a freedom fighter and you are winning the war.

Week Four - Day Five

Warm-Up for Week Four - Day Five

We're going to try something different and let each person call out a movement. Just be sure you start out slowly and build. Have fun with this. Someday when you are on vacation or for some other reason are away from the program you will realize that you've stored enough of it in your heart and minds that you can get in a workout and talk about the values that are important to you. This program will in time become a part of you and a part of your family.

To Share with the Family

This would be a good time for everyone to express thankfulness for the time the family has been spending together. This will be a special time full of memories and laughter. You may want to occasionally snap a few pictures during the workouts and if you do you can use them to remind you of all the happy times. Fifteen minutes doesn't sound like much but it does add up. The Saturday activities add even more because you took some extra time together.

Parent's Points to Ponder

Recently, I watched some geese make a home out of a flower pot in front of an office building. Geese have a reputation for fiercely defending their homes. When my oldest daughter, Jennifer, was two years old she innocently wandered too close to a goose at a petting zoo. We both quickly learned how ill-advised that was as I snatched her away from being pecked.

We can all learn a lesson from geese though. We need to fight to protect all aspects of the home life of our children. We need to bring some things in like healthy, whole foods and keep some things out like television programs that wreck havoc on their nervous system with graphic violence and inappropriate images.

Research has shown that when you watch images of something happening to someone of your same sex that your nervous system will react as though it was happening to you. Think before you watch a movie or something on television. Stress hormones tend to make us hold weight in the abdominal area.

What good are you hoping to gain from stressful images? Be a good gatekeeper of your children's minds and your own. Error on the side of preserving innocence. It will be gone soon enough.

Breakthrough Workout for Week Four - Day Five

Even on day five this week, I want you to purposely do fewer reps and sets. We'll start with lunges, then side planks, push-ups, and mountain climbers. If you like, you can do a reassessment of your upper body strength by doing as many push-ups as you can. This is optional but might reinforce that you are making progress every day.

Cool Down for Week Four - Day Five

Alternate walking and skipping. Slowly do some running arms. Stretch as you would when you first awake. Stretch until you feel great.

Character Classics

Talk about what it would be like to write the story of your family's life together. How would you be described in that book?

Character Challenge

Think about someone you'd like to call or see and then be sure to do it. Don't take friendships and family for granted. Find time to be hospitable with those you love.

Mom's Moment

Congratulations, champion! You are finishing your first month. Most months have a few extra days and that helps if for any reason we miss a day. They can also be used to repeat a day you really enjoyed or felt challenged by. There is no need to be rigid. Let the program fit your family.

If you work on the weekends and have time off during the week, you'll obviously want to adjust the schedule to fit those realities. Think about adjustments you'll want to make in month two. Order or design the next month's workouts. Bask in all that you've accomplished. This oasis of family love and support will have benefits for generations to come.

Saturday is Game Day

Big game day is a chance to really go all out. Our character quality this week is hospitality. Hospitality is being generously open to others and involves treating guests well. Game day is the perfect time to invite another family to do something active like skating, bowling or any other activity you would all enjoy. This is a day to celebrate the new lifestyle you have achieved by sticking with the program for a full month. Congratulations!

Sunday is Rest Day

Enjoy a day of rest and relaxation and get ready for next month and all the happiness your family will enjoy. You will find that by cutting back a little in the fourth week that you will be ready for new challenges in the next month. Recovery is vital to long term success.

This is also the perfect time to take stock of all that you have accomplished this month. The family time, the healthier choices, the activities, and the character growth all point to a job well done. This is the beginning of knowing that you are leading your family to increased health, fitness, and happiness. Well done!

Parenting with a Purpose

You have spent the last month with a clear set of goals for improving many aspects of your family life. You used your imagination and the power of association to make healthy choices desirable. Consider the influence you have had.

As you continue on this journey, I'd like to offer you continued support. There will be email updates and blog posts that I hope you find useful. In addition, by joining the monthly Exercising Values program, you will continue to have a full month of workouts, character qualities, and stories to use each month. I hope you visit www.exercisingvalues.com often. The blog is there to give you valuable new information and to help us keep in touch.

When you started your family, chose your career, or decided to homeschool, you probably had some end goal in mind no matter how vague. Over time, parts of that vision were clarified, reversed, or abandoned. As you progress with the Exercising Values program your goals will also develop. Feel free to contact me, via the website, with questions as they come up. I invite you to sign up and continue with the program you have started.

	Week One	Week Two
Character Quality	Enthusiasm	Loyalty
Warm-Up	Marching Front Kick Side Kick Back Kick Moon Reach Lawn Mower	Marching Front Kick Side Kick Back Kick Moon Reach Lawn Mower
Cardio	Mountain Climbers	Burpees
Upper Body	Push-Ups	Dips
Abs	Planks	Crunches
Lower Body	Lunges	One Leg Deadlifts
Cool-Down	Marching Front Kick Side Kick Back Kick Lawn Mower Moon Reach Partner Stretch	Marching Front Kick Side Kick Back Kick Lawn Mower Moon Reach Partner Stretch
Mom's Moment	Catch a Vision List Goals Acknowledge Contact Nap	Drink Water Rethink Diet Finish Plan Menus Enjoy Life
Literature	Tom Sawyer Pollyanna	Tom Sawyer Pollyanna
Character Challenge	Smile Influence Cheerful Work Build Enthusiasm	Participate Take Action Be Charitable

	Week Three	Week Four
Character Quality	Diligence	Hospitality
Warm-Up	Running Leaping Waving Shifting	Running Leaping Waving Shifting
Cardio	Jumping Jacks	Jumping Jacks
Upper Body	Running Arms	Running Arms
Abs	Partner Pull-Ups	Partner Pull-Ups
Lower Body	Squats	Squats
Cool-Down	Running Leaping Waving Shifting Top-To-Bottom Partner Stretch	Running Leaping Waving Shifting Top-To-Bottom Partner Stretch
Mom's Moment	Note Progress New Habits Act of Kindness	Connect
Literature	Tom Sawyer Pollyanna	Tom Sawyer Pollyanna
Character Challenge	Finish Projects	Demonstrate

Look at all you have accomplished!

Bask for just a moment in the joy of taking action and reaping results.

I'd love to hear about your progress. I can be reached at:

pamdavenport@exercisingvalues.com

For more help along your journey please visit my website:

www.exercisingvalues.com

Congratulations on a month of devotion to your family!

CPSIA information can be obtained at www.ICGtesting.com
Printed in the USA
LVOW10s1112261015

459771LV00001B/69/P